55 EMERGENCIES ONE MUST KNOW BEFORE 55

Dedicated to

MY MOTHER

G. SUFIA BI

Who was always a Poetess at Heart

ACKNOWLEDGEMENTS

This book would not have seen the light of the day, but for

My Father **Dr. B. Sheik Ali** who has an endless passion in the pursuit of education,

My Wife **Farheen** for shouldering newer responsibilities,

My Daughters **Zainab and Zeba Raisa** from whom I am still learning.

CHAPTERS

1. Shock — 8
2. Altered Mental status and Coma — 10
3. Choking — 12
4. Swallowed objects — 14
5. Asthma — 16
6. Pneumonia — 18
7. Sudden Respiratory Disorders in Children — 20
8. Pulmonary Edema — 22
9. Smoke Inhalation — 24
10. Palpitation — 26
11. Heart Attack — 28
12. Hypertensive Crises — 30
13. Pericarditis — 32
14. Stroke — 34
15. Meningitis — 36
16. Gastritis — 38
17. Hepatitis — 40
18. Gall Stones — 42
19. Haemorrhoids — 44
20. Gasrtoenteritis — 46
21. Appendicitis — 48
22. Melena — 50
23. Renal Stones — 52
24. Urinary Tract Infection — 54
25. Acute Retention of Urine — 56
26. Renal Failure — 58
27. Arthritis — 60
28. Near Drowning — 62

29. Electrical Injuries	64
30. Heat Illness	66
31. Alcohol Intoxication	68
32. Seizures in children	70
33. Poisons	72
34. Bites and Stings	74
35. Abortion	76
36. Eclampsia	78
37. Ectopic Pregnancy	80
38. Pelvic Inflammatory Disease	82
39. Testis Torsion	84
40. Acute Psychosis	86
41. Burns	88
42. Head Injury	90
43. Trauma to Neck	92
44. Upper Limb Injury	94
45. Lower Limb Injury	96
46. Chest Trauma	98
47. Pelvic Fractures	100
48. Eye Problems	102
49. Bleeding from the Nose	104
50. Dental Emergencies	106
51. Throat Emergencies	108
52. Diabetes	110
53. Thyroid Problems	112
54. Adrenal Problems	114
55. Skin Problems	116
IMPORTANT POINTS TO REMEMBER	118
INDEX	120
REFERENCES	124

> "A TEACHER TEACHES A LESSON AND GIVES A TEST, WHEREAS LIFE GIVES US A TEST WHICH TEACHES A LESSON"

(The author's favorite quote and also wants to put in writing that every EMERGENCY patient he has seen has taught him a lesson and hence is grateful to them)

GUIDE LINES IN USING THIS BOOK AND HOW ONE CAN BENEFIT FROM THIS BOOK

A Thought in every topic to keep one motivated

A simple line drawing but useful information

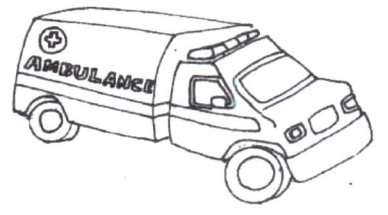

HOW TO IDENTIFY IT?

This box is colored red to signify its importance and early identification which can be critical.

HOW TO DEAL?

What one has to do when faced with a problem as from the red box. This is highlighted in yellow for one to be ready at any time.

WHAT WILL BE DONE IN THE HOSPITAL?

One is in a safe territory where emergencies will be handled but still one has to know what action will be taken there which is highlighted by green.

IMPORTANT AND ADVANCED INFORMATION

A blue colored highlighted box is for optional information and for those who want to know more.

1. SHOCK

" Most of us are about as eager to be changed as we were to be born, and go through our changes in a similar state of shock."-Aristotle

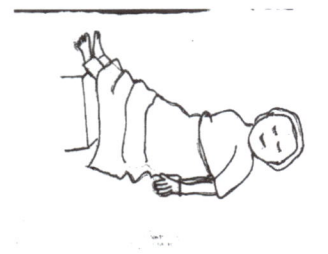

POSITIONING IN SHOCK

To keep the person warm and comfortable If neck injury is not suspected to turn the victim's head to one side

HOW TO IDENTIFY IT?
Signs of shock include:

1. Sudden loss of consciousness
2. Feeling very weak
3. Light headedness
4. Dizziness or giddiness
5. Unable to walk and less alert than normal

HOW TO DEAL?
- **STEP 1 Identification is most important. Take immediate action as one may be able to save a life. Call Ambulance service if one is not sure.**
NEVER LEAVE THE PERSON UNATTENDED.
- **STEP 2 Have the person lie down and check for any injury to the head and neck or chest and keep the legs flat. Otherwise raise the person's legs upwards on a box like structure for about 30 centimeters.**
- **STEP 3 If the person vomits, turn the person to one side to drain the fluids from the mouth as it can get into the lungs.**
- **STEP 4 Any obvious bleeding has to be controlled by pressure application and to note for any broken bones and to splint them if necessary.**
- **STEP 5 Repeated monitoring of the pulse is necessary to know the state of shock and always keep the person warm by wrapping with blanket.**

WHAT WILL BE DONE IN THE HOSPITAL?

Many actions will be taken simultaneously by hospital personnel in an EMERGENCY DEPARTMENT to stabilize the person in shock after an initial assessment of the person. The first course of action will be the assessment of ABC which are

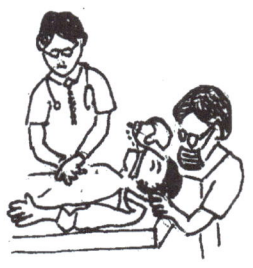

CARDIOPULMONARY RESUCSITATION

Airway: assessment will be done whether the person is awake enough to try to take their own breaths and/or if there anything blocking the mouth or nose.

Breathing: assessment of the adequacy of breathing will be done and decided whether it will need to be assisted with mouth-to-mouth resuscitation or more aggressive interventions like a bag and mask or intubation with an endotracheal tube.

Circulation: assessment of the adequacy of the blood pressure will be made and determined whether intravenous lines will be needed for delivery of fluid or medications to support the blood pressure.

Patients will be treated with oxygen supplementation through nasal cannulae, a face mask, or endotracheal intubation.

Blood will be transfused if bleeding is the cause of the shock state.

Further investigations will be requested to know the cause of shock such as Electrocardiogram, blood investigations and other imaging studies and once the cause is known, this will be treated immediately.

If the condition demands, the person will be further admitted in an Intensive Care unit of the Hospital or will be further observed and assessed.

IMPORTANT AND ADVANCED INFORMATION
COMMON CAUSES

Hypovolemic shock is the most common type of shock and is caused by insufficient circulating volume.[1] Its primary cause is hemorrhage (internal and/or external), or loss of fluid from the circulation. Vomiting and diarrhea are the most common cause in children.[2]

Cardiogenic shock is caused by the failure of the heart to pump effectively.[1] This can be due to damage to the heart muscle, most often from a large myocardial infarction. Other causes of cardiogenic shock include dysrhythmias, cardiomyopathy/myocarditis, congestive heart failure (CHF), or cardiac valve problems.[2]

Obstructive shock is due to obstruction of blood flow outside of the heart.[1] Several conditions can result in this form of shock which are Cardiac tamponade [2],Tension pneumothorax[2] ,Pulmonary embolism and Aortic stenosis

Distributive shock is due to impaired utilization of oxygen and thus production of energy by the cell.[1] Examples of this form of shock are:Septic shock

2. ALTERED MENTAL STATUS AND COMA

"It doesn't matter who you were or what you've done in the past. The only thing that matters is who you are right now." — Shelly Crane,

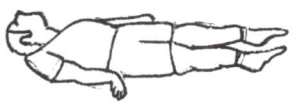

DECEREBERATE POSITION

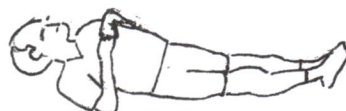

DECORTICATE POSITION

HOW TO IDENTIFY IT?

1. Sudden change in behavior.
2. Does not respond in a normal manner when previously was doing so.
3. Shows no response on repeated pinching.
4. Body st a stiff position without movement.
5. At times the person responds, but goes to an alterestered state.

HOW TO DEAL?

- **STEP1** Follow all the steps of Shock from 1 to 5 as on page 8 and with priority of maintenance of airway.
- **STEP 2** In case if the person has become comatose as a result of Diabetes, check for a quick blood glucose if available, follow instructions as specified by the attending doctor.
- **STEP 3** Watch for respiratory efforts and count the respiratory rate as this can give an idea of the state of person (Increased respiration can mean lack of oxygenation and decreased respiration can mean condition of person is deteriorating).
- **STEP 4** Start CPR (see Page 118)

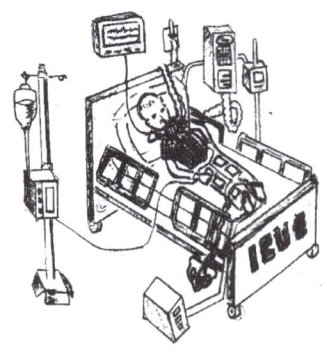
COMA MANAGEMENT

WHAT WILL BE DONE IN A HOSPITAL?

It is critical in all comatose patients to stabilize first and advanced life support system will be initiated if the person has been brought with continuous cardiopulmonary resuscitation.
Persons in either an altered mental status or a comatose state will be checked for a blood glucose value to rule out low blood glucose if not done earlier and intravenous glucose will be administered if it is low.

If breathing is irregular and respiratory functions showing deterioration with low oxygen values, the person will be immediately intubated to maintain sufficient oxygenation to the lungs.
At the same time if there is compromise in the circulatory state, intravenous fluids will be administered.
Blood will be collected for relevant investigations including for drug levels if suspected poisoning.
Other relevant investigations as in Shock stage such as ECG, X-rays or Ultrasound will also be requested
An Emergency CT Scan will be asked in all persistent coma stage where the cause is not known and in all cases of preceding head injuries
Subsequently the person if still in comatose stage will be admitted in an Intensive Care Unit for need of serial evaluation, observation and further management.

IMPORTANT AND ADVANCED INFORMATION
COMMON CAUSES
Coma may result from a variety of conditions, including intoxication (such as drug abuse, overdose or misuse of over the counter medications, prescribed medication, or controlled substances), metabolic abnormalities, central nervous system diseases, acute neurologic injuries such as strokes or herniations, hypoxia, hypothermia, hypoglycemia or traumatic injuries such as head trauma caused by falls or vehicle collisions. It may also be deliberately induced by pharmaceutical agents in order to preserve higher brain functions following brain trauma, or to save the patient from extreme pain during healing of injuries or diseases.[3]

3. CHOKING

> "Freedom is strangely ephemeral. It is something like breathing; one only becomes acutely aware of its importance when one is choking."
> ~William E. Simon

HEIMLICH MANEUVER

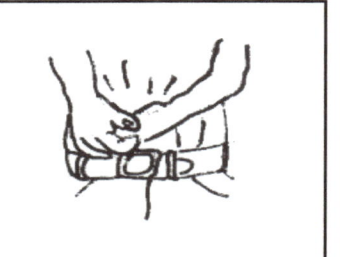

HOW TO DEAL?
Choking Rescue Procedure (Heimlich Maneuver) - Choking While Alone
- If one chokes when alone, fists must be used to do thrusts on oneself. Or one must lean over the back of a chair and pressed hard to pop out the object.

Choking Rescue Procedure (Heimlich Maneuver) - Baby (Younger Than 1 Year)
- If the baby can cough or make sounds, let him or her cough to try to get the object out. If one is worried about the baby's breathing, call 911.
  If a baby can't breathe, cough, or make sounds, then:
   Keep the baby's face down on one's forearm so the baby's head is lower than his or her chest.
- Support the baby's head in one's palm, against one's thigh and do not cover the baby's mouth or twist his or her neck.
  Use the heel of one's hand to give up to 5 back slaps between the baby's shoulder blades.
- If the object does not pop out, support the baby's head and turn him or her face up on one's thigh. Keep the baby's head lower than his or her body.
- Place 2 or 3 fingers just below the nipple line on the baby's breastbone and give 5 quick chest thrusts.
- Keep giving 5 back slaps and 5 chest thrusts until the object comes out or the baby faints.
- If the baby faints, call 911 (if one hasn't called already). Then:
- Do not do any more back slaps or chest thrusts.
- Start CPR. If one does rescue breaths, to look for an object in the mouth or throat each time the airway is opened during CPR. If one sees the object, it is taken out. But if one can't see the object, one's finger must not be stuck down the baby's throat to feel for it.
- Keep doing CPR until the baby is breathing on his or her own or until help arrives.

CHOKING RESCUE PROCEDURE

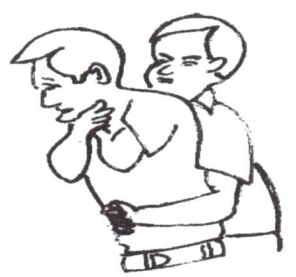

HOW TO DEAL?
Choking Rescue Procedure (Heimlich Maneuver) - Adult or Child Older Than 1 Year
- If the person can cough or make sounds, let him or her cough to try to get the object out. If one is worried about the person's breathing, call 911.
- If the person can't breathe, cough, or make sounds, then:

- Stand or kneel behind the person and wrap one's arms around his or her waist. If the person is standing, place one of the legs between his or her legs so one can support the person if he or she faints.
- Make a fist with one hand and place the thumb side of one's fist against the person's belly, just above the belly button but well below the breastbone.
- Grasp with the fist the other hand and give a quick upward thrust into the belly. This may cause the object to pop out. One may need to use more force for a large person and less for a child or small adult.
- Repeat thrusts until the object pops out or the person faints.
  Call 911 or other emergency services if the person faints. Then:
- Start CPR (cardiopulmonary resuscitation) if one knows how to do it.
- If one is doing rescue breaths, look for an object in the mouth or throat each time the airway is opened during CPR. The object is removed when seen.
- Do not do any more Heimlich thrusts.
- Keep doing CPR until the person is breathing on his or her own or until help arrives.

IMPORTANT AND ADVANCED INFORMATION
COMMON CAUSES
Respiratory diseases that involve obstruction of the airway.
Compression of the laryngopharynx, larynx or vertebrate trachea in strangulation.
Foreign bodies, but consisting of any object which comes from outside the body itself, including food, toys or household objects) in the airway.[4]
This type of choking is often suffered by small children, who are unable to appreciate the hazard inherent in putting small objects in their mouth.[5] In adults, it mostly occurs whilst the patient is eating.

4. SWALLOWED OBJECTS

"By swallowing evil words unsaid, no one has ever harmed his stomach."
Winston Churchill

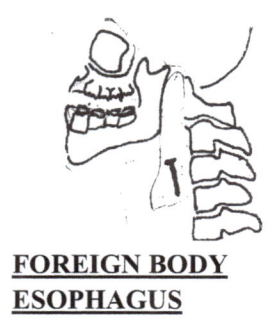

FOREIGN BODY ESOPHAGUS

HOW TO IDENTIFY IT?
1. There is history of swallowed objects.
2. Person unable to swallow later.
3. Stuck sensation in the upper food tube (esophagus).
4. At times persisitent vomiting and pain in the abdomen area.
5. Change in the colour of stools.

HOW TO DEAL?
- **STEP 1** Identification of the object which has been swallowed is important. Most of the objects which are harmless will usually come out of the stools and hence one has to observe the stools for he object.
- **STEP 2** However if the swallowed object gets stuck in the throat one has to see in the EMERGENCY DEPARTMENT for assessment.
- **STEP 3** Following objects which have been swallowed will need immediate consultation

    -poisonous substances like drugs, mushrooms

    -open pins, razor blades

    -metallic objects like nails, needles, wire

    -objects like marbles, plastic objects and the like

WHAT WILL BE DONE IN THE HOSPITAL?
An initial assessment will be made to determine the location of the swallowed foreign body. And in case if there is respiratory distress or abdominal complaints, relevant investigations will be asked such as X-ray, endoscopy, or barium swallow to help find the object if it doesn't come out in the stool, or if an inhaled object has not been coughed out.

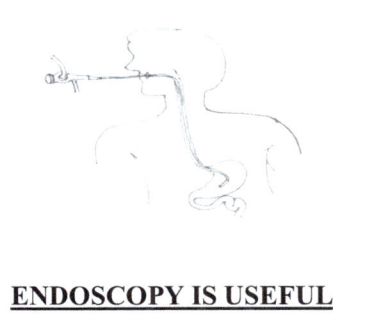

ENDOSCOPY IS USEFUL

A special metal detector will be used to locate a metallic object, such as a coin, inside the body. The doctor will then recommend a procedure such as the use of an Esophagoscope to remove the object or will simply encourage one to continue to observe the stools for the swallowed foreign object.

ADVANCED INFORMATION
COMMON CAUSES

The objects most commonly swallowed by children are coins.[6] Meat impaction is more common in adults.[7]

Swallowed objects are more likely to lodge in the esophagus or stomach than in the pharynx or duodenum.[8]

Swallowed batteries can be associated with additional damage,[10][11] with mercury poisoning (from mercury batteries) and lead poisoning (from lead batteries) presenting important risks.

One technique used is endoscopic foreign body retrieval.

Endoscopic retrieval involves the use of a gastroscope or an optic fiber charge-coupled device camera. This instrument is shaped as a long tube, which is inserted through the mouth into the esophagus and stomach to identify the foreign body or bodies. This procedure is typically performed under conscious sedation. Many techniques have been described to remove foreign bodies from the stomach and esophagus. Usually the esophagus is protected with an overtube (a plastic tube of varying length), through which the gastroscope and retrieved objects are passed.[12]

Once the foreign body has been identified with the gastroscope, various devices can be passed through the gastroscope to grasp or manipulate the foreign body. Devices used include forceps, which come in varying shapes, sizes and grips,[13] snares, and oval loops that can be retracted from outside the gastroscope to lasso objects,[14] as well as Roth baskets (mesh nets that can be closed to trap small objects),[15] and magnets placed at the end of the scope or at the end of orogastric tubes.[13][16] Some techniques have been described that use foley catheters to trap objects, or use two snares to orient foreign bodies.[9]

5. ASTHMA

> "For breath is life, and if you breathe well you will live long on earth." ~Sanskrit Proverb

NEVER UNDERESTIMATE ASTHMA. IT CAN BE DANGEROUS!!

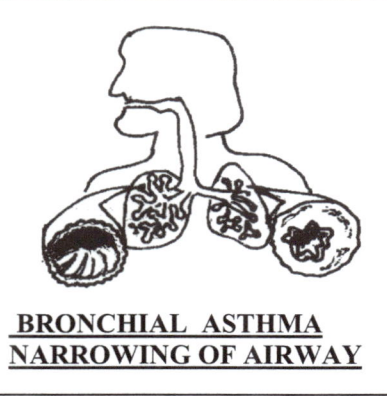

BRONCHIAL ASTHMA NARROWING OF AIRWAY

HOW TO IDENTIFY IT?
1. Persistent cough.
2. Breathlessness
3. Feeling of tightness of chest or chest pain
4. Increased respiratory efforts
5. At times lips, tongue, nails and bod can become blue and unable to complete sentences.

HOW TO DEAL?
- **STEP 1** Identification is important. Identify whether the asthma is mild moderate or severe. Severity will be known by the ability to speak, rate of respiration, breathing difficulty and ability to walk).
- **STEP 2** If asthmatic attack is severe call for an Ambulance service first and meanwhile give oxygen and nebulization if available.
- **STEP 3** If the asthmatic attack is moderate use an inhaler which would have been prescribed before or give nebulization with bronchodilators with the correct dosage and check for response.
- **STEP 4** If the asthmatic attack is mild, follow the Doctors instructions and keep a continuous observation.
- **STEP 5** It is important to remember that there can be a sudden change from moderate to severe.
- **STEP6** Develop an Asthma Action Plan by identifying
  -asthma triggers and subsequently to avoid them.
  -a list of peak flow meter readings and record the person's best readings for future use.
  -name and dose of asthma medications that need to be taken.

WHAT WILL BE DONE IN THE HOSPITAL?

The severity of the asthmatic attack will be assessed quickly. If in severe respiratory distress, simultaneous oxygen will be given with nebulization with drugs causing opening of the airways (called as Bronchoilators) and will be monitored

If person does not show considerable improvement, arterial blood gas estimation will be done and depending on the values, after proper sedation if necessary ,a tube will be put in the airway (endotracheal intubation), mechanical ventilation will be done.

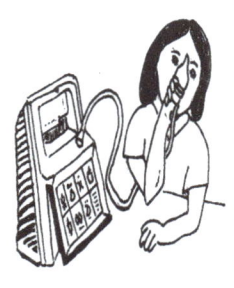

NEBULIZATION

At the same time steriods will also be administered and the hydration status will be corrected if necessary. Person will be subsequently admitted in an ICU for frequent evaluation and observation.

In case of moderate degree of asthma, oxygen along with nebulization and steroids as above will be given and observed. Improvement will be assessed by using a device called a peak flow meter which will show how quickly the air is exhaled from the lung. Person will be discharged if considerable improvement after observation for some time.

IMPORTANT AND ADVANCED INFORMATION
COMMON CAUSES
Environmental
Many environmental factors have been associated with asthma's development and exacerbation including: allergens, air pollution, and other environmental chemicals.[17]
Genetic
Family history is a risk factor for asthma with many different genes being implicated.[18]
Medical conditions
A triad of atopic eczema, allergic rhinitis and asthma is called atopy.[19] with asthma occurring at a much greater rate in those who have either eczema or hay fever.[20]
Beta blocker medications such as propranolol can trigger asthma in those who are susceptible.[21] Other medications that can cause problems are ASA, NSAIDs, and angiotensin-converting enzyme inhibitors.[22]
Exacerbation
Home factors that can lead to exacerbation of asthma include dust, animal dander (especially cat and dog hair), cockroach allergens and mold.[23]
Both viral and bacterial infections of the upper respiratory tract can worsen the disease.[23]

6. PNEUMONIA

"Never forget that it is not a pneumonia, but a pneumonic man who is your patient." Medscape

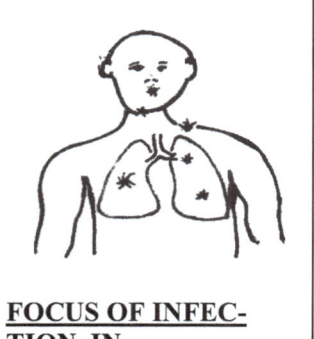

FOCUS OF INFECTION IN PNUEMONIA

HOW TO IDENTIFY IT ?
1. Bad cough with purulent sputum, many times greenish.
2. High fever.
3. Tightness of chest wall and chest pain.
4. Increased respiratory efforts like increased breathing.
5. At times lips, tongue and nails can become blue.

HOW TO DEAL?
STEP 1 If one has identified the person to have Pneumonia, That person has to be taken to the EMERGENCY DEPARTMENT for further care.
STEP 2 Initially if the fever is high, Paracetamol can be given (see dosage page119). Suspected Pneumonia must never be dealt at home.

WHAT WILL BE DONE IN THE HOSPITAL ?
A preliminary diagnosis of Pneumonia will be made after a detailed examination, especially of the respiratory system and with relevant investigations such as X-rays and blood investigations.

Blood investigations which will be necessary is for culture and sensitivity in order to isolate the organism and its effectiveness to antibiotics.

The person with Pneumonia will be monitored and oxygen will be given if necessary along with antipyretics, correction of hydration and antibiotics commenced where considered necessary.

At times in case of severe bilateral pneumonia or acute respiratory distress syndrome (ARDS), ventilation with low tidal volumes (6ml/Kg body weight) will be required and these persons will be admitted in an Intensive care unit for further observation.

In other cases where a diagnosis of Pneumonia has been made and its cause known and the condition is satisfactory will be asked for proper follow up and discharged.

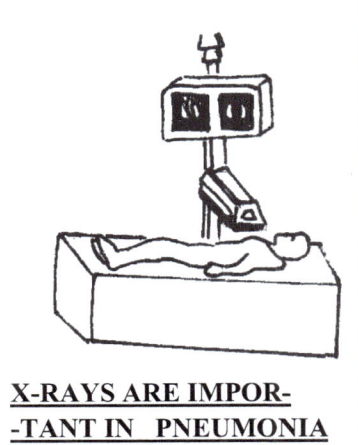
**X-RAYS ARE IMPOR-
-TANT IN PNEUMONIA**

IMPORTANT AND ADVANCED INFORMATION
COMMON CAUSES
Bacteria

Bacteria are the most common cause of community-acquired pneumonia (CAP), with *Streptococcus pneumoniae* isolated in nearly 50% of cases.[24] Other commonly isolated bacteria include: *Haemophilus influenzae Chlamydophila pneumoniae* i and *Mycoplasma pneumoniae* ;[24] *Staphylococcus aureus*; *Moraxella catarrhalis*; *Legionella pneumophila* and Gram-negative bacilli.[25]

A number of drug-resistant versions of the above infections are becoming more common, including drug-resistant *Streptococcus pneumoniae* (DRSP) and methicillin-resistant Staphylococcus aureus (MRSA).[26]

Viruses

Commonly implicated agents include: rhinoviruses, coronaviruses, influenza virus, respiratory syncytial virus (RSV), adenovirus, and parainfluenza.[27][28] Herpes simplex virus rarely causes pneumonia, except in groups such as: newborns, persons with cancer, transplant recipients, and people who have significant burns.[29]

Fungi

Fungal pneumonia is uncommon, but occur more commonly in individuals with weakened immune systems due to AIDS, immunosuppressive drugs, or other medical problems.[30] It is most often caused by *Histoplasma capsulatum*, blastomyces, *Cryptococcus neoformans*, *Pneumocystis jiroveci*, and *Coccidioides immitis*.

Parasites

A variety of parasites can affect the lungs, including: *Toxoplasma gondii*, *Strongyloides stercoralis*, *Ascaris lumbricoides*, and *Plasmodium malariae*.[31] These organisms typically enter the body through direct contact with the skin, ingestion, or via an insect vector.[31]

Idiopathic

Idiopathic interstitial pneumonia or noninfectious pneumonia[32] are a class of diffuse lung diseases. They include: diffuse alveolar damage, organizing pneumonia, nonspecific interstitial pneumonia, lymphocytic interstitial pneumonia, desquamative interstitial pneumonia, respiratory bronchiolitis interstitial lung disease, and usual interstitial pneumonia.[33]

7. SUDDEN RESPIRATORY DISORDERS IN CHILDREN

"When you own your breath, nobody can steal your peace." - Puranas

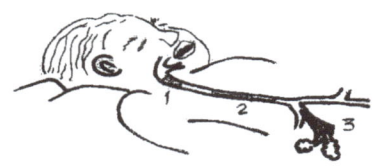

1. EPIGLOTITIS
2. CROUP
3. BRONCHIOLITIS

HOW TO IDENTIFY IT ?
1. Cough which sounds like barking type.
2. Breathing which is very noisy.
3. Increased respiratory efforts like increased breathing
4. Fever at times, not feedinf well or persistent vomiting.
5. Can become bluish.

HOW TO DEAL ?
Always seek expert care if one is not confident in handling. Proceed to the EMERGENCY DEPARTMENT if child is in distress.

HOME REMEDIES FOR CROUP
- STEP 1 Steam therapy is very helpful. Hold the child in one's arms near the steam source (taking proper precautions about the source) and expose to 20 to 30 minutes.
- STEP 2 See for the degree of response. If not responding well and if in any doubt proceed to the nearest EMERGENCY DEPARTMENT.
- STEP3 Always check for the temperature and give Paracetamol in correct dosage if having fever (See page 119). This will bring down the temperature and lower the respiratory rate.
- STEP 4 Give plenty of oral fluids to prevent dehydration.
- STEP 5 Avoid precipitating factors like cigarette smoke, dust, dirt or pollen grains

WHAT WILL BE DONE IN THE HOSPITAL ?
The degree of respiratory distress will be assessed initially. A correct diagnosis will be made depending on the presentation. If the symptoms are severe enough, the child will be given inhaled medications such as racemic epinephrine in the emergency room. Other treatment will involve the use of humidified oxygen and frequent nebulization and observation.

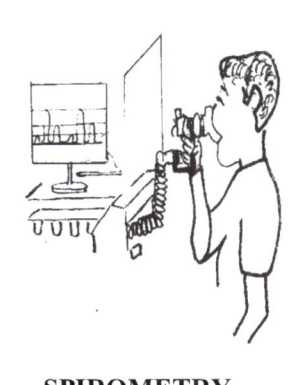
SPIROMETRY

At times if the child is in severe distress with low oxygen values will require ventilation which will be done by experts in the field. They will also require nasogastric tubes to assist in ventilation. Intensive monitoring will be done and necessary investigations will be requested in an Intensive Care unit.
In case of croup Dexamethasone (medication belonging to steroid group) will be given X-rays will also be requested and in case of suspected bacterial infection, antibiotics will be administered.

IMPORTANT AND ADVANCED INFORMAT
COMMON CAUSES

Croup is usually deemed to be due to a viral infection.[34][35] Others use the term more broadly, to include acute laryngotracheitis, spasmodic croup, laryngeal diphtheria, bacterial tracheitis, laryngotracheobronchitis, and laryngotracheobronchopneumonitis. The first two conditions involve a viral infection and are generally milder with respect to symptomatology; the last four are due to bacterial infection and are usually of greater severity.[36]

Stridor may occur as a result of:
Foreign bodies (e.g., aspirated peanut, aspirated food bolus);
Tumor (e.g., laryngeal papillomatosis, squamous cell carcinoma of larynx, trachea or esophagus);
Infections (e.g., epiglottitis, retropharyngeal abscess, croup);
Subglottic stenosis (e.g., following prolonged intubation or congenital);
Airway edema (e.g., following instrumentation of the airway, tracheal intubation, drug side effect, allergic reaction);
Subglottic hemangioma (rare);
Vascular rings compressing the trachea;
Many thyroiditis such as Riedel's thyroiditis;
Vocal cord palsy;
Tracheomalacia or Tracheobronchomalacia (e.g., collapsed trachea).
Congenital anomalies of the airway are present in 87% of all cases of stridor in infants and children.[36]
Vasculitis.

Epiglottitis involves bacterial infection of the epiglottis, most often caused by Haemophilus influenzae type B, although some cases are attributable to *Streptococcus pneumoniae, Streptococcus agalactiae, Staphylococcus aureus, Streptococcus pyogenes, Haemophilus influenzae*, and *Moraxella catarrhalis*.

8. PULMONARY EDEMA

"Breath is the bridge which connects life to consciousness, which unites your body to your thoughts." ~Thick Nhat Hanh

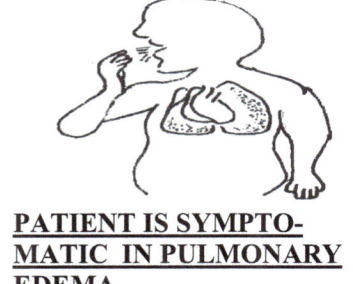

PATIENT IS SYMPTOMATIC IN PULMONARY EDEMA

HOW TO IDENTIFY IT ?
1. Sudden breathlessness.
2. Very bad cough, cannot lie down.
3. Chest pain with sweating at times.
4. Increased respiratory efforts
5. Feels extremely weak and has difficulty in walking.

HOW TO DEAL ?
- **Proceed to the nearest EMERGENCY DEPARTMENT if one is experiencing difficulty in breathing and bad cough.**
- **Pulmonary Edema can be life threatening and must be treated in a Hospital.**

WHAT WILL BE DONE IN THE HOSPITAL?

Pulmonary edema will be considered as an Acute emergency and will be treated urgently.

The airway is checked to be clear and high flow oxygen with face mask will be given.

Medications such as diuretics (water pills) will be administered intravenously.

If considerable distress morphine will also be given along with an antiemetic (medication to stop vomiting).

The patient will be monitored for urine output and if required will be admitted in an Intensive Care Unit.

The treatment for noncardiac causes of pulmonary edema varies depending on the cause. If severe infection (sepsis) is suspected it will be treated with antibiotics and other supportive measures.

In case of kidney failure evaluation and further management of the initial cause will be carried out.

At times invasive monitoring such as urinary, intraarterial, central venous and Swan-Ganz catheter will be required.

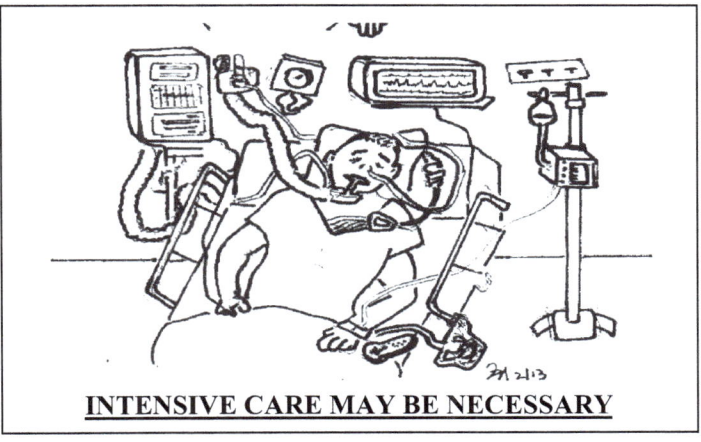

INTENSIVE CARE MAY BE NECESSARY

IMPORTANT AND ADVANCED INFORMATION
COMMON CAUSES
Cardiogenic
Left ventricular failure may be due to a heart attack leading to arrhythmias (tachycardia/fast heartbeat or bradycardia/slow heartbeat) and fluid overload, e.g., from kidney failure or intravenous therapy which may cause dilatation and failure of the left ventricle or may cause pulmonary edema in the absence of heart failure.

Non-cardiogenic
Hypertensive crisis. Upper airway obstruction (negative pressure pulmonary edema[37])
Neurogenic causes[38] (seizures, head trauma, strangulation, electro

Other/unknown
Injury to the lung may also cause pulmonary oedema through injury to the vasculature and parenchyma of the lung. The acute lung injury-acute respiratory distress syndrome (ALI-ARDS) covers many of these causes, but they may include:
Inhalation of hot or toxic gases
Pulmonary contusion, i.e., high-energy trauma (e.g. vehicle accidents)
Aspiration, e.g., gastric fluid
Reexpansion, i.e. post large volume thoracocentesis, resolution of pneumothorax, post decortication, removal of endobronchial obstruction, effectively a form of negative pressure pulmonary oedema.
Reperfusion injury, i.e. postpulmonary thromboendartectomy or lung transplantation
Immersion pulmonary edema[39][40]
Multiple blood transfusions
Severe infection or inflammation which may be local or systemic. This is the classical form of ALI-ARDS.

9. SMOKE INHALATION

"Unbeknownst to many people, smoke inhalation actually remains the number one cause of death from indoor fires." Medscape

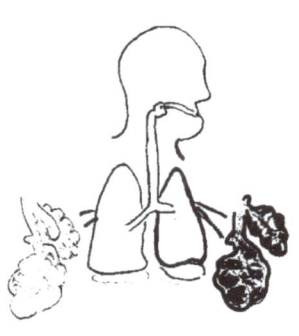

SMOKE PARTICLES IN DISTAL ALVEOLI

HOW TO IDENTIFY IT?

1. History of exposure to smoke
2. Increased respiratory efforts with breathing difficulties
3. At times can see soot in the nostrils
4. Very bad cough and difficulty in speaking.
5. Sore throat.

HOW TO DEAL?
STEP 1. Move the person to safety.
STEP 2 Assess the gravity of situation.
STEP 3 Start CPR (see page118) if necessary.
STEP 4 If person in state of shock adopt Step 1 to Step 5 as in Shock stage (See page 8)
STEP 5 Continuous observation is important. All smoke inhalation persons have to be evaluated in an EMERGENCY DEPARTMENT

WHAT WILL BE DONE IN THE HOSPITAL?

The extent of smoke inhalation will be assessed and if the person is in a state of severe respiratory distress will be handled if necessary with mechanical ventilation by means of endotracheal intubation. Visualization by means of upper and lower airway with fiberoptic bronchoscope will also be considered.

In case of moderate degree of respiratory distress arising from smoke inhalation, bronchodilators will be given along with parenteral antibiotics.

In case of mild cases , observation will be done to see for any later developments of respiratory distress or its complications and treated.

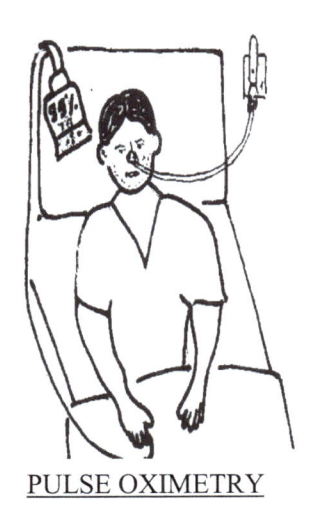

PULSE OXIMETRY

IMPORTANT AND ADVANCED INFORMATION
COMMON CAUSES
Smoke inhalation injury, either by itself but more so in the presence of body surface burn, can result in severe lung-induced morbidity and mortality.[41] The most common cause of death in burn centers is now respiratory failure. Injury to the lungs and airways is not only due to deposition of fine particulate soot but also due to the gaseous components of smoke which include phosgene, carbon monoxide and sulfur dioxide.

10. PALPITATION

Hold fast to your dreams, for without them life is a **broken** winged bird that cannot fly." Langston Hughes

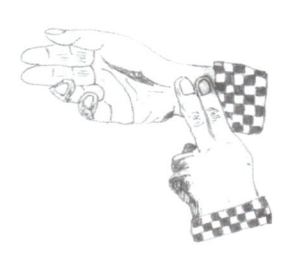

PALPITATION CAN BE DETECTED BY COUNTING THE HEART RATE

HOW TO IDENTIFY IT ?
1. Feels heart is beating very fast.
2. At times breathing difficulty.
3. Giddiness and feeling of discomfort.
4. Chest pain and sweating at times with back pain.
5. Unable to sleep and vomiting at times.

HOW TO DEAL ?
- **STEP 1** If one feels uncomfortable with the above symptoms seek help in an **EMERGENCY DEPARTMENT**.
- **STEP 2** If person is on the verge of collapse, follow Steps as in Shock on page 8.
- **STEP 3** If person is already on medication or on any new medications for other conditions, make sure that this medication is taken to the hospital.
- **STEP 4** If one is confident about the cause of palpitation and seen earlier and evaluated and the medication has been deferred, this should be looked into and taken as advised.
- **STEP 5** Long standing palpitation must never be neglected as this can affect the heart.

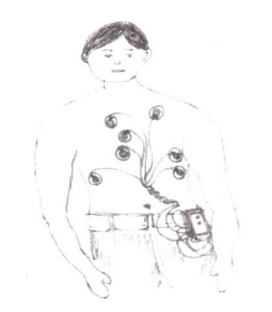

HOLTER MONITORING IS HELPFUL IN ANALYSING THE HEART RATE

WHAT WILL BE DONE IN THE HOSPITAL?

Initially the general condition of the person will be assessed and if not in shock or severe respiratory distress an Electrocardiogram will be done and the exact cause ascertained.

Further treatment depends on the rate of heart beat. If it is very rapid and more than 200/minute, medications known as Lignocaine or Adenosine will be given intravenously and constantly monitored for the degree of response.

In case where palpitation is from other causes such as thyroid problem or high fever, this will be corrected with proper respective medications. Persons who are in severe respiratory distress will be monitored in an Intensive Care set up.

Further imaging studies will be done such as ECHO, CAT scan or scintillation studies will be done along with blood investigations for cardiac functions.

At times pace maker will be considered necessary when no shown enough response with medications.

IMPORTANT AND ADVANCED INFORMATION
COMMON CAUSES

Palpitations can be attributed to one of three main causes:

Hyperdynamic circulation (valvular incompetence, thyrotoxicosis, hypercapnia, pyrexia, anemia, pregnancy).

Sympathetic overdrive (panic disorders, hypoglycemia, hypoxia, levocetirizine antihistamines, anemia, heart failure, mitral valve prolapse).[42]

Cardiac dysrhythmias (premature atrial contraction, junctional escape beat, premature ventricular contraction, atrial fibrillation, supraventricular tachycardia, ventricular tachycardia, ventricular fibrillation, heart block). Anxiety can also cause palpitations in that the heart muscles are affected by the state of one's mind. Psychological problems can thus induce one to palpitate.

11. HEART ATTACK

"The most important thing in illness is never to lose heart." ~Nikolai Lenin

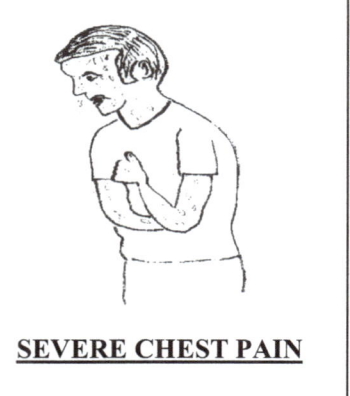

SEVERE CHEST PAIN

HOW TO IDENTIFY IT ?
1. Very severe chest pain with sweating.
2. Radiating pain to the left arm and at times to the jaw and neck.
3. At times breathing difficulties.
4. Pain in the upper part of abdomen.
5. Vomiting may be present at times.

HOW TO DEAL ?
- **STEP 1** If one suspects a heart attack call the Ambulance service immediately as time is critical.
- **STEP 2** If person is in Shock, follow Steps as in Shock on page 8
- **STEP 3** Awareness is equally important and mild symptoms like indigestion, fatigue or stress must not be neglected.
- **STEP 4** Mild symptoms can be just as serious and life threatening of heart attack that causes severe chest pain. Hence one has to proceed to an EMERGENCY DEPARTMENT, especially the elderly people and persons with risk factors such as high blood pressure, diabetics, people with kidney problems and with heart problems.

WHAT WILL BE DONE IN THE HOSPITAL?
Once the person arrives in the EMERGENCY DEPARTMENT an urgent Electrocardiogram will be done to confirm the heart attack.
Supplemental oxygen to increase the supply of oxygen to the heart's muscle will be given at once along with strong pain killers mainly morphine and this will be given in titrated doses depending on the level of response. Medications called GTN will be given either in patch form or underneath the tongue if blood pressure is stable.

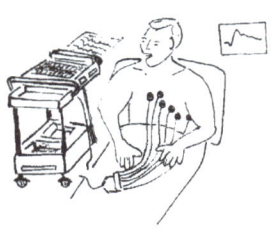
ELECTROCARDIOGRAM

Soluble aspirin will also be given provided there is no allergy to it
Anti-platelet medications to prevent formation of blood clots in the arteries will be administered.
Medications to decrease the need for oxygen by the heart's muscle and to prevent abnormal heart rhythms will also be administered.

Coronary angiography with either percutaneous transluminal coronary angioplasty (PTCA) with or without stenting to open blocked coronary arteries wherever facilities are available will be carried out.
All persons with a heart attack will be monitored in the Intensive Coronary Unit for further observation and management.

IMPORTANT AND ADVANCED INFORMATION

Myocardial infarction results from atherosclerosis.[43]
Risk factors for myocardial infarction include:
Age[44]
Gender: At any given age men are more at risk than women, particularly before menopause,[45] but because in general women live longer than men ischemic heart disease causes slightly more total deaths in women.[10]
Diabetes mellitus (type 1 or 2)[46]
High blood pressure[47]
Dyslipidemia/hypercholesterolemia (abnormal levels of lipoproteins in the blood), particularly high low-density lipoprotein, low high-density lipoprotein and high triglycerides[47]
Tobacco smoking, including secondhand smoke[47]
Short term exposure to air pollution including: carbon monoxide, nitrogen dioxide, and sulfur dioxide but not ozone.[48]
Family history of ischaemic heart disease or myocardial infarction particularly if one has a first-degree relative (father, brother, mother, sister) who suffered a 'premature' myocardial infarction (defined as occurring at or younger than age 55 years (men) or 65 (women).[44]
Obesity[49] (defined by a body mass index of more than 30 kg/m², or alternatively by waist circumference or waist-hip ratio).
Lack of physical activity.[44]
Alcohol — Studies show that prolonged exposure to high quantities of alcohol can increase the risk of heart attack.
Oral contraceptive pill – women who use combined oral contraceptive pills have a modestly increased risk of myocardial infarction, especially in the presence of other risk factors, such as smoking.[50]

12. HYPERTENSIVE CRISES

"I took everything with a pinch of salt and now I've hypertension." Unknown

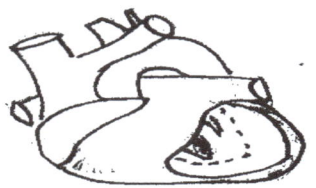

HYPERTENSIVE HEART THICKENING IN WALL OF VENTRICLES

HOW TO IDENTIFY IT?
1. Bad headache may be present.
2. Blurring of vision.
3. At times chest pain.
4. Shotness of breath.
5. Swelling of the lower limbs.

HOW TO DEAL?
- **STEP1 Serial measurement of blood pressure is important. If blood pressure readings are high and identified to be in the potentially dangerous readings one must proceed to the EMERGENCY DEPARTMENT as organ damage can occur.**
- **STEP 2 if person has defaulted medication, taking the antihypertensive medications at the proper time and dosage is important and must be emphasized to prevent crises.**

WHAT WILL BE DONE IN THE HOSPITAL ?
Initially the Blood Pressure (BP) will be checked in all extremities with an appropriately sized BP cuff, and pulses will be assessed in all extremities.
In a hypertensive emergency, the first goal will be to bring down the blood pressure as quickly as possible with intravenous (IV) blood pressure medications to prevent further organ damage The drug of choice will depend on the clinical situation.
The person will be put on exogenous oxygen depending on O_2 saturation levels or arterial blood gas results, continuous cardiac monitoring will be done.
An indwelling arterial line will have to be inserted at times.
Examination of the eye is considered important to look for swelling and bleeding. Whatever organ damage that has occurred will be treated with therapies specific to the organ that is damaged.
Person will be observed and managed if necessary in an Intensive Care unit.

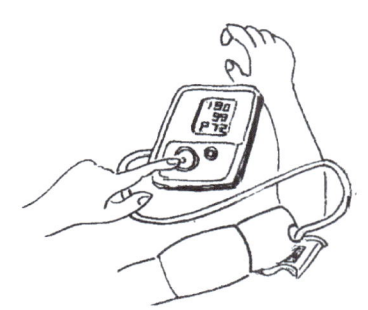

SERIAL EVALUATION OF BLOOD PRESSURE IS IMPORTANT

IMPORTANT AND ADVANCED INFORMATION
COMPLICATIONS

The eyes may show retinal hemorrhage or an exudate. Papilledema must be present before a diagnosis of malignant hypertension can be made.

The brain shows manifestations of increased intracranial pressure, such as headache, vomiting, and/or subarachnoid or cerebral hemorrhage.

Patients will usually suffer from left ventricular dysfunction.

The kidneys will be affected, resulting in hematuria, proteinuria, and acute renal failure.

It differs from other complications of hypertension in that it is accompanied by papilledema.[51] This can be associated with hypertensive retinopathy.

DRUGS USED

Several classes of antihypertensive agents are recommended, with the choice depending on the etiology of the hypertensive crisis, the severity of the elevation in blood pressure, and the usual blood pressure of the patient before the hypertensive crisis.

In most cases, the administration of an intravenous sodium nitroprusside injection, which has an almost immediate antihypertensive effect, is suitable (but in many cases not readily available). In less urgent cases, oral agents like captopril, clonidine, labetalol, or prazosin can be used, but all have a delayed onset of action (by several minutes) compared to sodium nitroprusside.

It is also important that the blood pressure be lowered smoothly, not too abruptly. The initial goal in hypertensive emergencies is to reduce the pressure by no more than 25% (within minutes to 1 or 2 hours), and then toward a level of 160/100 mm Hg within a total of 2–6 hours. Excessive reduction in blood pressure can precipitate coronary, cerebral, or renal ischemia and, possibly, infarction.[52]

The diagnosis of a hypertensive emergency is not based solely on an absolute level of blood pressure, but also on the typical blood pressure level of the patient before the hypertensive crisis occurs. Individuals with a history of chronic hypertension may not tolerate a "normal" blood pressure.

13. PERICARDITIS

"A cheerful heart is good medicine, but a crushed spirit dries up the bones." (Proverbs 17:22)

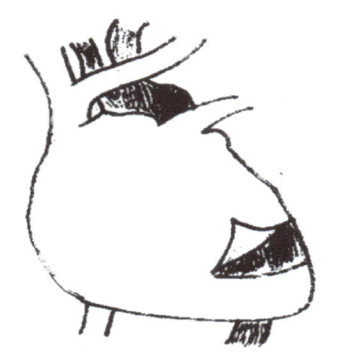

PERICARDIIUM FILLED WITH FLUID

HOW TO IDENTIFY IT?
1. Chest pain and more when taking deep breath.
2. Pain in the chest becoming more when lying down flatand better when leaning forward.
3. At times pain in the upper part of the abdomen.
4. Pain when swallowing at timed may be present.
5. Associated fever or cough.

HOW TO DEAL?
- **STEP 1 If person is experiencing following symptoms and signs as specified above, proceed to the nearest EMERGENCY DEPARTMENT.**
- **STEP 2 This is life threatening and correct identification is important which can be done only in a hospital.**
- **STEP 3 Follow up also will be equally important till complete recovery.**

WHAT WILL BE DONE IN THE HOSPITAL?
Initial diagnosis will be made by use of Electrocardiogram (ECG), ECHO and other investigations.

Primary treatment will be relief of pain and this will be initiated by use of anti-inflammatory medications such as Ibubrufen. Narcotic pain medications such as Codeine or Morphine will have to be used at times.

The cause of pericarditis will be determined by means of further investigations.

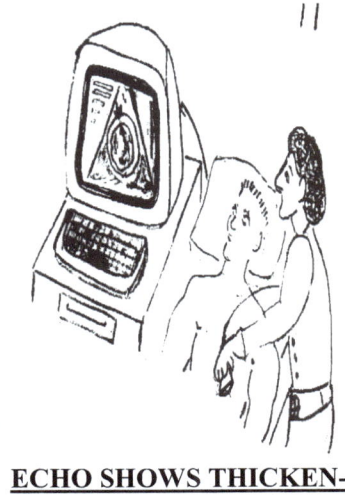

ECHO SHOWS THICKENING OF PERICARDIUM

Use of corticosteroids will also be considered in case of immunological compromised persons or recurrent pericarditis.

If fluid is detected in the pericardial sac, a procedure known as pericardiocentesis will be done. This will involve inserting a thin needle into the pericardial sac and aspirating out the pericardial fluid.

Other procedures involve Pericardiotomy and Pericardectomy where the former procedure involve cutting a hole in the pericardial sac and the latter involve removing the pericardial sac. These procedures will be done by experts in their field.

IMPORTANT AND ADVANCED INFORMATION
COMMON CAUSES
Infectious

Pericarditis may be caused by viral, bacterial, or fungal infection. The most common viral pathogen has traditionally been considered to be coxsackievirus based on studies in children from the 1960s, but recent data suggest that adults are most commonly affected with cytomegalovirus, herpesvirus, and HIV.[53][54] Pneumococcus or tuberculous pericarditis are the most common bacterial forms. Anaerobic bacteria can also be rare cause.[55] Fungal pericarditis is usually due to histoplasmosis, or in immunocompromised hosts Aspergillus, Candida, and Coccidioides. The most common worldwide cause of pericarditis is infectious pericarditis with Tuberculosis.

Others

Idiopathic: No identifiable etiology found after routine testing.
Immunologic conditions including systemic lupus erythematosus (more common among women) or rheumatic fever
Myocardial Infarction (Dressler's syndrome)
Trauma to the heart, e.g. puncture, resulting in infection or inflammation
Uremia (uremic pericarditis)
Malignancy (as a paraneoplastic phenomenon)
Side effect of some medications, e.g. isoniazid, cyclosporine, hydralazine, warfarin, and heparin
Radiation induced
Aortic dissection
Tetracyclines
Postpericardiotomy syndrome: Usually after CABG surgery

14. STROKE

"I do not believe that any man fears to be dead, but only the stroke of death."- Francis Bacon

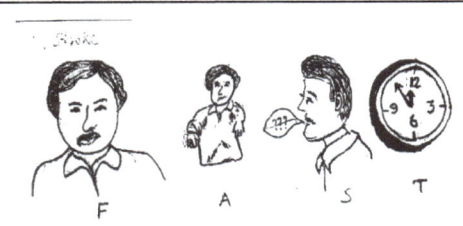

FACE: Smile Is one side droopy?
ARMS: Raise Is one side weak?
SPEAK: Is it slurred?
TIME: Lost time could be lost brain

HOW TO IDENTIFY IT?
1. Sudden weakness in one half of the body or in both upper limbs.
2. Not able to speak properly.
3. Drooling from the mouth.
4. Not able to walk.
5. At times severe headache and visual problems.

HOW TO DEAL?
- STEP 1 If person is in a state of shock follow steps as in shock page
- STEP 2 If person in coma follow steps as on page 10.
- STEP 3 If one has symptoms of stroke like and they go away, it must not be neglected and assessment is equally important in a Hospital set up as this can be from a condition known as Transcient Ischemic Attack (TIA) which may be a precursor of stroke. Early treatment for TIA can help to prevent stroke.

WHAT WILL BE DONE IN THE HOSPITAL?
Initially the person will be examined in detail with emphasis on neurological evaluation and confirmation of a stroke.
Vital signs will be recorded and stabilization will be initiated if necessary
This involves oxygen therapy, airway maintenance and control of blood pressure. An emergency CT scan will be requested and the cause whether it is Ischemic or Hemorrahagic will be determined.
Simultaneously symptomatic treatment will be carried for relief of headache, the hydration status will be considered and if necessary a feeding tube will be put in the stomach.
Once the stroke is confirmed to be from a clot, clot-busting drugs (thrombolytic therapy) will be used. These blood thinners commonly used will be heparin or warfarin. Aspirin or clopidogrel (Plavix) will also be used if necessary.

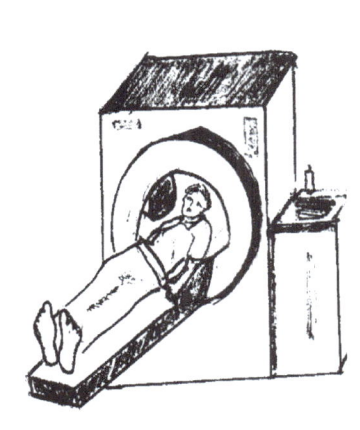

CT SCAN IS A MUST

In case of confirmed Hemorrhagic stroke, person will be handled by Neurosurgeon for need of further management. This may involve removing the blood around the brain or to repair damaged blood vessels.

Advanced surgical procedures such as surgery on carotid artery will also be considered where necessary.

All patients with stroke will have to be subjected to swallowing therapy, physical therapy, speech therapy and occupational therapy depending on the extent of stroke.

IMPORTANT AND ADVANCED INFORMATION
COMMON CAUSES

Thrombotic stroke
In thrombotic stroke a thrombus[56] (blood clot) usually forms around atherosclerotic plaques. Since blockage of the artery is gradual, onset of symptomatic thrombotic strokes is slower.

Embolic stroke
An embolic stroke refers to the blockage of an artery by an arterial embolus, a travelling particle or debris in the arterial bloodstream originating from elsewhere. An embolus is most frequently a thrombus, but it can also be a number of other substances including fat (e.g., from bone marrow in a broken bone), air, cancer cells or clumps of bacteria (usually from infectious endocarditis).

Systemic hypoperfusion
Systemic hypoperfusion is the reduction of blood flow to all parts of the body. It is most commonly due to heart failure from cardiac arrest or arrhythmias, or from reduced cardiac output as a result of myocardial infarction, pulmonary embolism, pericardial effusion, or bleeding.

Intracerebral hemorrhage
It generally occurs in small arteries or arterioles and is commonly due to hypertension, intracranial vascular malformations (including cavernous angiomas or arteriovenous malformations), cerebral amyloid angiopathy, or infarcts into which secondary haemorrhage has occurred.[57] Other potential causes are trauma, bleeding disorders, amyloid angiopathy, illicit drug use (e.g., amphetamines or cocaine). The hematoma enlarges until pressure from surrounding tissue limits its growth, or until it decompresses by emptying into the ventricular system, CSF or the pial surface. A third of intracerebral bleed is into the brain's ventricles.

15. MENINGITIS

"It would be better to err in seeing a doctor and finding out it is not meningitis than to wait and find out it is." Medscape

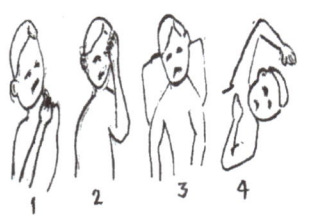

SYMPTOMS OF MENINGITIS
1. STIFF NECK
2. HEADACHE
3. DROWSINESS
4. FITTING

HOW TO IDENTIFY IT?
1. Bad headache
2. Neck pain or stiffness.
3. Vomiting
4. At times fever and restlessness
5. Seizures (abnormal movements) can occur at times.

HOW TO DEAL?
- **STEP 1** Meningitis can be potentially dangerous and hence a correct diagnosis is important. In the event of a person having the above symptoms proceed to an EMERGENCY DEPARTMENT.
- **STEP 2** Presence of a maculopapular rash with fever and neck stiffness is life threatening and has to be treated immediately. Seek EMERGENCY care.
- **STEP 3** Home treatment is only for diagnosed cases of Viral Meningitis who are stable. They will need proper hydration care with oral fluids and medications for pain care as prescribed earlier. Follow up is also important.

WHAT WILL BE DONE IN THE HOSPITAL?
Initially a diagnosis of meningitis has to be confirmed. This will include a detailed clinical examination with presence of neck rigidity and other clinical parameters. A lumbar puncture for collection of cerebrospinal fluid will be done and sent to the laboratory for analysis.

A person who has severe meningitis will be treated in the intensive care unit (ICU) of a hospital for observation and further management.

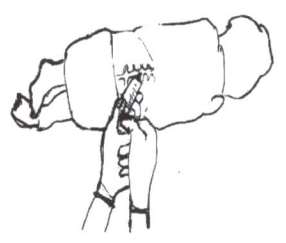

SPINAL TAPPING FOR CONFIRMATION

In case of confirmed bacterial meningitis, intravenous antibiotics in proper high doses and according to the hospital policy will be administered

If meningitis is causing pressure within the brain, corticosteroid medicines such as dexamethasone will be given to adults or children.

Medicines such as acetaminophen (Tylenol), will also be given to reduce fever.

If one has seizures, medications such as phenobarbital or Dilantin will be given to control seizures.

Oxygen therapy will also be considered if one has trouble breathing and to increase the amount of oxygen in all parts of the body.

Fluids will be monitored and given into a vein (IV) if one has an infection and is vomiting or is unable to drink enough. Doctors will also control the amount of fluids given because people with meningitis may develop problems if they have too much or not enough fluid.

Blood chemicals will be monitored and frequent blood tests will be done to measure essential body chemicals, such as sodium and sugar in the blood.

IMPORTANT AND ADVANCED INFORMATION
COMMON CAUSES

Meningitis is typically caused by an infection with microorganisms. Most infections are due to viruses,[58] with bacteria, fungi, and protozoa being the next most common causes.[59] It may also result from various non-infectious causes. [59] The term *aseptic meningitis* refers to cases of meningitis in which no bacterial infection can be demonstrated. This type of meningitis is usually caused by viruses, but it may be due to bacterial infection that has already been partially treated, when bacteria disappear from the meninges, or pathogens infect a space adjacent to the meninges (e.g. sinusitis). Endocarditis (an infection of the heart valves which spreads small clusters of bacteria through the bloodstream) may cause aseptic meningitis. Aseptic meningitis may also result from infection with spirochetes, a type of bacteria that includes *Treponema pallidum* (the cause of syphilis) and *Borrelia burgdorferi* (known for causing Lyme disease). Meningitis may be encountered in cerebral malaria (malaria infecting the brain) or amoebic meningitis, meningitis due to infection with amoebae such as *Naegleria fowleri*, contracted from freshwater sources.[59]

16. GASTRITIS

"To array a man's will against his sickness is the supreme art of medicine."
Sushruta

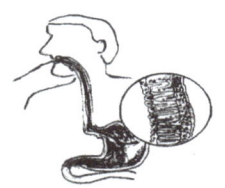

INFLAMMATION OF GASTRIC MUCOSA

HOW TO IDENTIFY IT?
1. Pain upper part of abdomen.
2. Vomiting.
3. Loss of appetite.
4. At times change in colour of stools.
5. Feeling of bloating sensation in the stomach.

HOW TO DEAL?
- **STEP 1** If one is sure it is gastritis, antacids available over the counter pharmacy can be taken with watchful observation.
- **STEP 2** If no improvement and pain increases one has to proceed to the nearest EMERGENCY DEPARTMENT for need of further evaluation and assessment.
- **STEP 3** If gastritis is better, even then follow up is essential in order to rule out some type of infections most common being Helicobacter type where doctors will prescribe specific medications which have to be taken.
- **STEP 4** Watchful waiting is important and in case of altered stool colour, especially blackish, one must proceed to the EMERGENCY DEPARTMENT to rule out any bleeding.
- **STEP 5** follow up and dietary guide lines will have to be strictly adhered to.

WHAT WILL BE DONE IN THE HOSPITAL
Initially a diagnosis of Gastritis will be made clinically taking into consideration a complete history and a physical examination.
If the gastritis is severe medications will be administered by parenteral means (intravenous or intramuscular) such as Antispasmodics or Proton Pump Inhibitors. If no significant improvement the following will be done

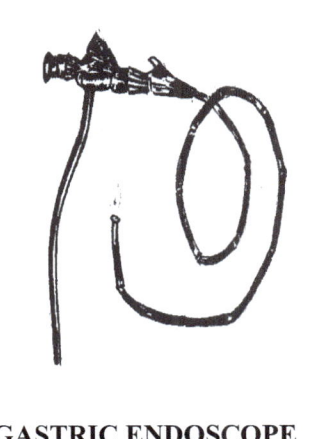
GASTRIC ENDOSCOPE

Blood tests. To see if there is any infective process going on. Also to see the extent of Hemoglobin to rule out any anemia Stool will be tested to detect if there is any blood in it which will give an idea of any bleeding going on in the gastrointestinal tract.

Upper Endoscopy A thin tube with a small camera attached to it will be inserted through the stomach to visualize its lining and to see if there is any associated inflammation. A small sample from the lining will be taken for need of further assessment .

IMPORTANT AND ADVANCED INFORMATION
COMMON CAUSES

Acute

Erosive gastritis is a gastric mucosal erosion caused by damage to mucosal defenses.[60]

NSAIDs inhibit cyclooxygenase-1, or COX-1, an enzyme responsible for the biosynthesis of eicosanoids in the stomach, which increases the possibility of peptic ulcers forming.[61] Also, NSAIDs, such as aspirin, reduce a substance that protects the stomach called prostaglandin. These drugs used in a short period are not typically dangerous. However, regular use can lead to gastritis.[62]

Chronic

Chronic gastritis refers to a wide range of problems of the gastric tissues.[60] The immune system makes proteins and antibodies that fight infections in the body to maintain a homeostatic condition. In some disorders the body targets the stomach as if it were a foreign protein or pathogen; it makes antibodies against, severely damages, and may even destroy the stomach or its lining.[62]
. Gastritis may also be caused by other medical conditions, including HIV/AIDS, Crohn's disease, certain connective tissue disorders, and liver or kidney failure.[63]

Helicobacter pylori colonizes the stomach of more than half of the world's population, and the infection continues to play a key role in the pathogenesis of a number of gastroduodenal diseases. Colonization of the gastric mucosa with *Helicobacter pylori* results in the development of chronic gastritis in infected individuals, and in a subset of patients chronic gastritis progresses to complications (e.g., ulcer disease, gastric neoplasias, some distinct extra-gastric disorders).[64]

17. HEPATITIS

"A disease known is half cured."
Hippocartus

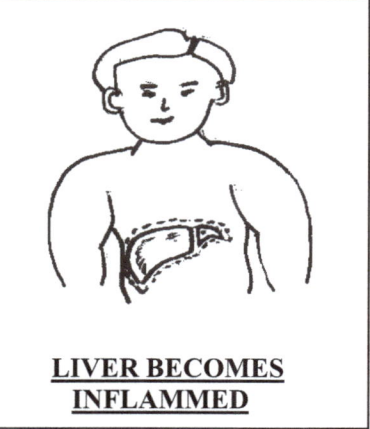

LIVER BECOMES INFLAMMED

HOW TO IDENTIFY IT?
1. Change in colour of skin or conjunctiva.
2. Dark coloured urine
3. Pain abdomen more on right side.
4. Loss of appetite.
5. At times nausea and vomiting.

HOW TO DEAL?
- **STEP 1** If person is experiencing bad pain abdomen with passing high colored urine, yellowish discoloration of skin and conjunctiva, proceed to the EMERGENCY DEPARTMENT for need of further evaluation and assessment.
- **STEP 2** If associated high fever, drug consumption or has received blood transfusion earlier and the person has above symptoms, it is important to seek EMERGENCY care.
- **STEP 3** Person who has already been diagnosed as having Hepatitis and if at home and develops altered sensorium or goes into coma, follow as in steps of Coma page 10.

WHAT WILL BE DONE IN THE HOSPITAL

The person will be examined for the general condition and seen for enlargement and tenderness of the liver along with presence of any free fluid in the abdomen.

If diagnosed as liver failure, very aggressive treatment will be necessary which will need stabilization if person is in shock (see SHOCK on page 9) monitoring of serum glucose and intracranial pressure. Fluid from the abdomen will be drained if excessive fluid is causing distress.

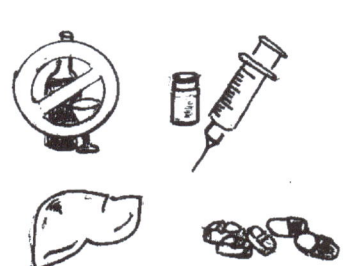

TREATMENT
STOP ALCOHOL
INTERFERON
LIVER TRANSPLANT
NEW MEDICATIONS IN FUTURE

Investigations will also be carried out to know the cause of Hepatitis and also its functioning capacity such as Hepatitis virus serologies Liver function tests Autoimmune blood markers Abdominal Ultrasound and Liver Biopsy

Further treatment will depend on the cause and will be initiated by Experts in that field.

IMPORTANT AND ADVANCED INFORMATION
COMMON CAUSES
Acute
Viral hepatitis
Bacterial
Protozoal
Parasitic
Fungal
Algal
Non infectious
Alcohol[65]
Auto immune conditions: systemic lupus erythematosus[66]
Drugs: Paracetamol, amoxycillin, antituberculosis medicines, minocycline and many others
Ischemic hepatitis (circulatory insufficiency)
Metabolic diseases: Wilson's disease[67]
Pregnancy
Toxins: Amanita toxin in mushrooms, carbon tetrachloride, asafetida
Chronic
Alcohol[65]
Autoimmune example Autoimmune hepatitis
Drugs examplesIsoniazid, Ketoconazole, Methyldopa, Nitrofurantoin
Inherited examples Wilson's disease[67] ,Alpha 1-antitrypsin deficiency
Non-alcoholic steatohepatitis
Viral hepatitis: (Hepatitis A does not cause chronic hepatitis)
Hepatitis B with or without hepatitis D, Hepatitis C, Hepatitis E[68]

18. GALL STONES

"It is a wise man's part to avoid sickness rather than to wish for medicines" Chinese proverb

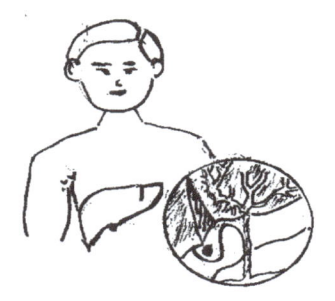

STONE IN THE GALL BLADDER

HOW TO IDENTIFY IT?
1. Pain abdomen right side.
2. Nausea and vomiting
3. Pain at times in the right shoulder blade
4. Change in the colour of stools at times
5. Loss of appetite or aversion to certain types of food.

HOW TO DEAL?
- **STEP 1** If person is experiencing persisting pain right side of abdomen with vomiting seek assistance in EMERGENCY DEPARTMENT for need of further evaluation and assessment.
- **STEP 2** Watchful waiting may be necessary at times.
- **STEP 3** If recurrent pain, associated yellowish discoloration of skin and conjunctiva and passing clay colored stools, at times will need Emergency Surgical Care.
- **STEP 4** If gall stones do not cause symptoms, careful observation will be sufficient.

WHAT WILL BE DONE IN THE HOSPITAL
A diagnosis of gall stones will be made initially by examination with presence of tenderness in the gall bladder area and with relevant investigations. If pain is significant pain killers will initially be given which can include opioids for relief. Simultaneously blood investigations and ultrasound will be requested.
Ultrasound is very useful as this will show the gall stones and the thickening of the gall bladder wall, presence of any fluid in it or any inflammation.

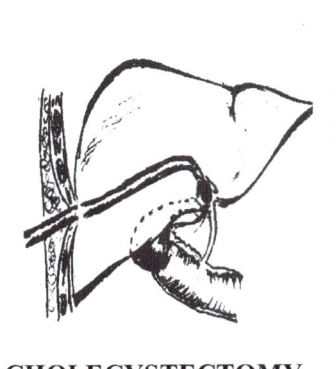

CHOLECYSTECTOMY

If person is having recurrent attacks of pain and there is no considerable relief surgery will be resorted to.
This will be done by means of laparoscopy where the gall bladder is removed by means of a small incision in the abdomen. In case of complicated cases will require an opening of the abdomen and further exploration.
For mild to moderate cases treatment includes bowel rest, intravenous fluids and antibiotics given through a vein with adequate pain relief medications.

IMPORTANT AND ADVANCED INFORMATION
COMMON CAUSES

Gallstone risk increases for females (especially before menopause) and for people near or above 40 years;[69]
A lack of melatonin could significantly contribute to gallbladder stones, as melatonin inhibits cholesterol secretion from the gallbladder, enhances the conversion of cholesterol to bile, and is an antioxidant, which is able to reduce oxidative stress to the gallbladder.[70] Researchers believe that gallstones may be caused by a combination of factors, including inherited body chemistry, body weight, gallbladder motility (movement), and perhaps diet. The absence of such risk factors does not, however, preclude the formation of gallstones.

Other nutritional factors that may increase risk of gallstones include rapid weight loss; constipation; eating fewer meals per day; and low intake of the nutrients folate, magnesium, calcium, and vitamin C.[71] On the other hand, wine and whole-grained bread may decrease the risk of gallstones.[72]. Risk factors for pigment stones include hemolytic anemias (such as sickle-cell disease and hereditary spherocytosis), cirrhosis, and biliary tract infections.[73] People with erythropoietic protoporphyria (EPP) are at increased risk to develop gallstones.[74][75] Additionally, prolonged use of proton pump inhibitors has been shown to decrease gallbladder function, potentially leading to gallstone formation.[76]

19. HAEMORRHOIDS

"Constipation is the best friend of hemorrhoids." Anonymous

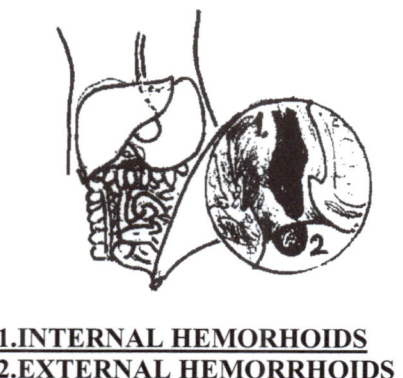

1. INTERNAL HEMORHOIDS
2. EXTERNAL HEMORRHOIDS

HOW TO IDENTIFY IT?
1. Persistent itching and uncomfortable sensation in the rectum.
2. Feeling of mass coming out when passing stools.
3. Blood usually fresh seen in the stools.
4. Pain when passing stools.
5. A hard painful mass can be felt at times.

HOW TO DEAL?
- **THIS DEPENDS UPON THE EXTENT**
- **STEP 1 If bleeding per rectum is profuse, person has to proceed to EMERGENCY DEPARTMENT for necessary evaluation and care.**
- **STEP 2 If external hemorrhoids are not very painful and relatively small, dietary fiber intake has to be increased along with increased water intake (provided there is no other associated heart, kidney or other problems where water intake has to be measured and taken) and prevent constipation.**
- **STEP 3 Itching sensation at the site can be lessened by application of creams or ointments available at over the counter pharmacy.**

WHAT WILL BE DONE IN THE HOSPITAL?
If there has been profuse bleeding per rectum and person is in shock stage will be treated as per SHOCK on page .

After stabilization and if the internal hemorrhoids is severe, surgery will be necessary.

The doctor will tie off the hemorrhoids with rubber bands or scar the tissue around the hemorrhoids. These treatments will reduce the blood supply to the hemorrhoids so that they shrink or go away.

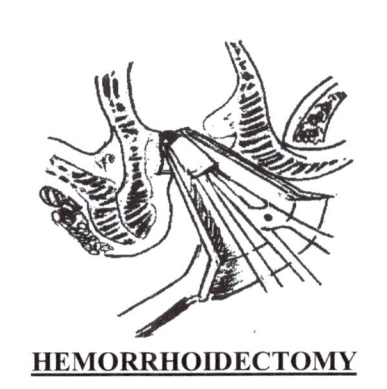
HEMORRHOIDECTOMY

In other symptomatic cases, an initial history taking and physical examination will reveal the extent of hemorrhoids which can also be known by examination with a lighted scope (instrument) inside the rectum. Oral medications and local applications will be prescribed.

IMPORTANT AND ADVANCED INFORMATION
COMMON CAUSES

The exact cause of symptomatic hemorrhoids is unknown.[77]

A number of factors are believed to play a role including: irregular bowel habits (constipation or diarrhea), a lack of exercise, nutritional factors (low-fiber diets), increased intra-abdominal pressure (prolonged straining, ascitis, an intra-abdominal mass, or pregnancy), genetics, an absence of valves within the hemorrhoidal veins, and aging.[78][79] Other factors that are believed to increase the risk include obesity, prolonged sitting,[80] a chronic cough and pelvic floor dysfunction.[81]

During pregnancy, pressure from the fetus on the abdomen and hormonal changes cause the hemorrhoidal vessels to enlarge. Delivery also leads to increased intra-abdominal pressures.[82] Pregnant women rarely need surgical treatment, as symptoms usually resolve after delivery.[78]

20. GASTROENTERITIS

"Whatever is on the floor will wind up in the baby's mouth. Whatever is in the baby's mouth will wind up on the floor." Medscape

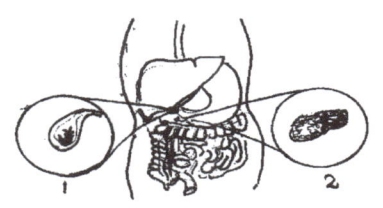

1. GALL BLADDER AND 2. PANCREAS CAN INVOLVE IN GASTROENTERITIS

HOW TO IDENTIFY IT?
1. Persistent diarrhea.
2. Vomiting which can be from few to many times.
3. Passing less amount of urine.
4. Feeling thirsty at times.
5. Dry mouth.

HOW TO DEAL?
- **STEP 1** IF signs of dehydration are severe as can be known by a look from a dry tongue, dry skin, eye balls shrunken and less amount of urination, one must seek help in the EMERGENCY DEPARTMENT.
- **STEP 2** Dehydration occurs faster in children than in adults and hence constant observation is very important. Meanwhile they must be given oral rehydration solutions in case if they are not vomiting which are easily available.
- **STEP 3** After every stool passed the oral rehydration solution should be given as tolerated preferably 1 to 3 ounces (30 to 90 ml) in children below 2 years and 3 to 8 ounces (90 to 240 ml) in older children and as much as possible in adults.
- **STEP 4** The brat diet which consists of Banana, Rice, Apple Sauce without sugar and Toast can be commenced as well.

WHAT WILL BE DONE IN THE HOSPITAL?

Initially the extent of dehydration will be assessed, whether it is mild, moderate or severe. If it is severe as evidenced by dry tongue, shrunken eye balls, less skin turgor or less amount of urination, immediate intravenous fluids will be commenced and relevant investigations will be carried out.

If gastroenteritis is of long standing duration, person will be evaluated by other specialists such as Gastroenterologist, Toxicologist or Surgeon.

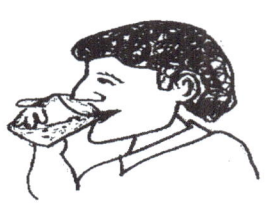

REHYDRATION IS IMPORTANT IN G.E.

In case of moderate dehydration, management will be on observation basis. Intravenous fluids will be started if not able to tolerate orally.

Mild dehydrated cases will be treated symptomatically with oral rehydration salts to be taken with water and for constant observation. Bowel binding agents are usually discouraged.

IMPORTANT AND ADVANCED INFORMATION
COMMON CAUSES

Viral

Rotavirus, norovirus, adenovirus, and astrovirus are known to cause viral gastroenteritis.[83][84] Rotavirus is the most common cause of gastroenteritis in children,[85] and produces similar incidence rates in both the developed and developing world.[86] Viruses cause about 70% of episodes of infectious diarrhea in the pediatric age group.[87] Rotavirus is a less common cause in adults due to acquired immunity.[88]

Bacterial

If food becomes contaminated with bacteria and remains at room temperature for a period of several hours, the bacteria multiply and increase the risk of infection in those who consume the food.[89] Some foods commonly associated with illness include raw or undercooked meat, poultry, seafood, and eggs; raw sprouts; unpasteurized milk and soft cheeses; and fruit and vegetable juices.[90] Toxigenic *Clostridium difficile* is an important cause of diarrhea that occurs more often in the elderly.[89] Infants can carry these bacteria without developing symptoms.[89] It is a common cause of diarrhea in those who are hospitalized and is frequently associated with antibiotic use.[91] "Traveler's diarrhea" is usually a type of bacterial gastroenteritis. Acid-suppressing medication appears to increase the risk of significant infection after exposure to a number of organisms, including *Clostridium difficile*, *Salmonella*, and *Campylobacter* species.[92] The risk is greater in those taking proton pump inhibitors than with H2 antagonists.[92]

Parasitic

A number of protozoans can cause gastroenteritis – most commonly *Giardia lamblia* – but *Entamoeba histolytica* and *Cryptosporidium* species have also been implicated.[87]

Non-infectious

There are a number of non-infectious causes of inflammation of the gastrointestinal tract.[93] Some of the more common include medications (like NSAIDs), certain foods such as lactose (in those who are intolerant), and gluten (in those

21. ACUTE APPENDICITIS

"He who has health has hope; and he who has hope has everything."
~Arabic Proverb

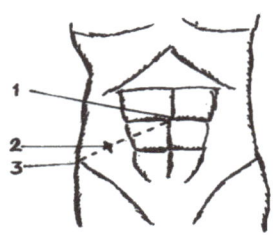

1. UMBILICUS
2. APPENDIX LOCATION
3. UPPER PART OF PELVIC BONE

HOW TO IDENTIFY IT?

1. Pain abdomen.
2. Persistent vomiting.
3. Feels feverish.
4. At times there can be diarrhea or pain when passing urine.
5. At times walks holding the abdomen on the right side.

HOW TO DEAL?

- **If one has one or all of the above complaints the person must be immediately consulted with a doctor to rule out appendicitis since a delay in seeking treatment will have an adverse outcome.**

WHAT WILL BE DONE IN THE HOSPITAL?

A diagnosis of Acute Appendicitis will usually be first made clinically and at times in doubtful cases will be confirmed by an Ultrasound examination.

Blood investigations will be asked for and in women of child bearing age group pregnancy will also be ruled out by a urine examination In case if the person is dehydrated Intra venous fluids will be commenced.

Analgesics (pain killer) and antiemetics (medication to control vomiting) will be administered. At times preoperative antibiotics intravenously will be administered.

Subsequently the patient will be evaluated by the Surgeon and appendicectomy (removal of the appendix) will be done.

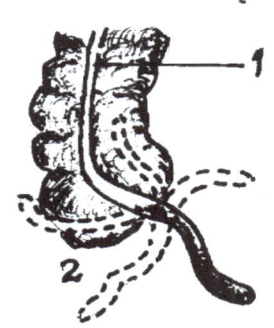

1. Tenia coli
2. VARIATIONS IN APPENDIX POSITION

IMPORTANT AND ADVANCED INFORMATION

On the basis of experimental evidence, acute appendicitis seems to be the end result of a primary obstruction of the appendix lumen (the inside space of a tubular structure).[94][95] Once this obstruction occurs, the appendix subsequently becomes filled with mucus and swells, increasing pressures within the lumen and the walls of the appendix, resulting in thrombosis and occlusion of the small vessels, and stasis of lymphatic flow.

Rarely, spontaneous recovery can occur at this point. As the former progresses, the appendix becomes ischemic and then necrotic. As bacteria begin to leak out through the dying walls, pus forms within and around the appendix (suppuration). The end result of this cascade is appendiceal rupture (a 'burst appendix') causing peritonitis, which may lead to septicemia and eventually death.

The causative agents include foreign bodies, trauma, intestinal worms, lymphadenitis, and, most commonly, calcified fecal deposits known as appendicoliths or fecaliths[96] The occurrence of obstructing fecaliths has attracted attention since their presence in patients with appendicitis is significantly higher in developed than in developing countries,[97] and an appendiceal fecalith is commonly associated with complicated appendicitis.[98] Also, fecal stasis and arrest may play a role, as demonstrated by a significantly lower number of bowel movements per week in patients with acute appendicitis compared with healthy controls.[99] The occurrence of a fecalith in the appendix seems to be attributed to a right-sided fecal retention reservoir in the colon and a prolonged transit time.[100] From epidemiological data, it has been stated that diverticular disease and adenomatous polyps were unknown and colon cancer exceedingly rare in communities exempt from appendicitis.[101][102] Also, acute appendicitis has been shown to occur antecedent to cancer in the colon and rectum.[103] Several studies offer evidence that a low fiber intake is involved in the pathogenesis of appendicitis.[104][105][106] This is in accordance with the occurrence of a right-sided fecal reservoir and the fact that dietary fiber reduces transit time.[107]

22. MELENA

"A pint of sweat will save a gallon of blood."-F.Bacon

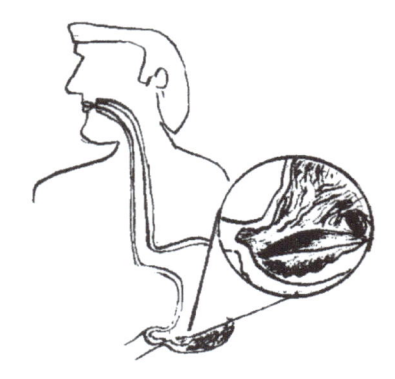

BLEEDING FROM THE STOMACH

HOW TO IDENTIFY IT?
1. Passing black coloured stools.
2. Pain abdomen, at times severe.
3. Person at times can appear pale.
4. Feels weak
5. At times blood can be seen in the stools which can be sticky and smells

HOW TO DEAL?
- **STEP 1 One must seek urgent consultation if one notices blood or change in the color of stools in the EMERGENCY DEPARTMENT.**
- **STEP 2 In children a small amount of blood may be seen in the stool. This again has to be evaluated to know the cause which could most probably be from milk allergy or long standing constipation.**

WHAT WILL BE DONE IN THE HOSPITAL?
The doctor will take a medical history and perform a physical examination, focusing on the abdomen and rectum. Treatment will depends on the cause and severity of the bleeding. Emergency treatment will include a blood transfusion. A nasogastric tube will be put and if there is massive bleeding, one will be monitored in an intensive care unit.

The following diagnostic tests will also be performed to know the cause of bleeding:

Ultrasound of the abdomen,
Angiography studies,
Barium studies,

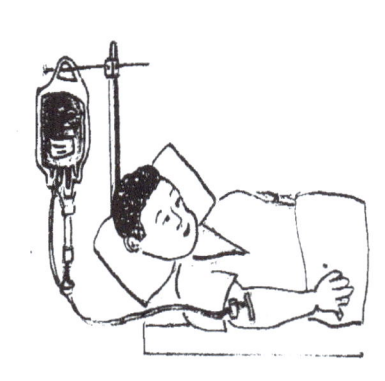
BLOOD TRANSFUSION

Blood studies, including a complete blood count and differential count, serum chemistries, clotting studies,
Colonoscopy,
Esophagogastroduodenoscopy or EGD,
Stool culture,
Tests for the presence of *Helicobacter pylori* infection,
X-rays of the abdomen
Esophagogastroduodenoscopy (EGD),
Radionuclide scanning.

Often endoscopy will be used to inject chemicals into the site of bleeding, or will treat the bleeding site with an electric current or laser, or apply a band or clip to close the bleeding vessel. If endoscopy does not control bleeding, the doctor will use angiography to inject medicine into the blood vessels to control bleeding. A last resort will be opening of the abdomen by a Surgeon and detect the bleeding source and control it (laporotomy).

IMPORTANT AND ADVANCED INFORMATION
COMMON CAUSES

The most common cause of melena is peptic ulcer disease. Any other cause of bleeding from the upper gastro-intestinal tract, or even the ascending colon, can also cause melena. Melena may also be a sign of drug overdose if a patient is taking anti-coagulants, such as warfarin. It is also caused by tumors, especially malignant tumors affecting the esophagus, more commonly the stomach & less commonly the small intestine due to their bleeding surface. However, the most prominent and helpful sign in these cases of malignant tumours is haematemesis. It may also accompany hemorrhagic blood diseases (e.g. purpura & hemophilia). Other medical causes of melena include bleeding ulcers, gastritis, esophageal varices, and Mallory-Weiss syndrome.

Causes of "false" melena include iron supplements, Pepto-Bismol, Maalox, and lead, blood swallowed as a result of a nose bleed (epistaxis), and blood ingested as part of the diet, as with consumption of black pudding (blood sausage), or with the traditional African Maasai diet, which includes much blood drained from cattle.

A less serious, self-limiting case of melena can occur in newborns two to three days after delivery, due to swallowed maternal blood.[108]

23. RENAL STONES

"Declare the past, diagnose the present, foretell the future." Hippocrates

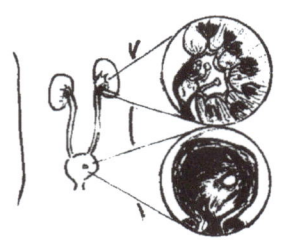

STONE IN THE CALYX & IN URINARY BLADDER

HOW TO IDENTIFY IT?
1. Pain abdomen radiating to the back at times.
2. Excruciating persistent pain and at times diddiculty in urination.
3. Passing high coloured urine.
4. At times fever and chills.
5. Nausea and vomiting.

HOW TO DEAL?
- **STEP 1** Renal stones at times cause severe pain in the back, abdomen or groin which at times will not be relieved by oral pain killers and will have to be handled in the EMERGENCY DEPARTMENT.
- **STEP 2** Water intake has to be increased in order to flush the stones taking into consideration that the person does not suffer from any other ailment.
- **STEP 3** Dietary modification will be necessary at times where the cause of stone formation is known which has to be followed as specified by the concerned specialist in care.

WHAT WILL BE DONE IN THE HOSPITAL?
This depends on the severity of pain caused by renal stones. After a cursory examination pain relief will be given and in case of severe pain opioids will be administered along with intravenous fluids.

Person will be subjected to further investigations such as Ultrasound or other imaging studies to see the status of kidney and the kidney stones.

Other diagnostic procedures which are helpful are intravenous pyelogram and ureteroscope.

Lithotripsy, which uses high-energy shock waves will also help to break up stones, and will be considered.

On confirmation of calcium oxalate stones, the doctor will prescribe a thiazide diuretic which prevents recurrences by decreasing the excretion of urine.

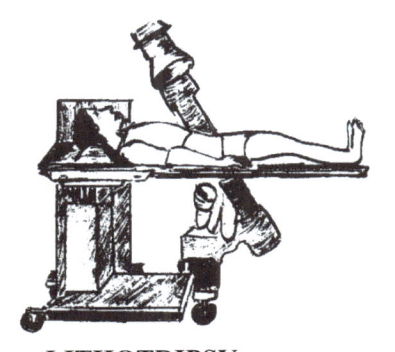
LITHOTRIPSY

Nephrolithotomy, will be the last resort for the removal of stone which uses a thin instrument that will be is inserted through an incision in the back. This procedure is done in most of the tertiary hospitals and will need frequent evaluation later .

IMPORTANT AND ADVANCED INFORMATION
COMMON CAUSES
Calcium-containing stones
By far, the most common type of kidney stones worldwide contains calcium Factors that promote the precipitation of oxalate crystals in the urine, such as primary hyperoxaluria, are associated with the development of calcium oxalate stones.[109] The formation of calcium phosphate stones is associated with conditions such as hyperparathyroidism[110] and renal tubular acidosis.[111]

Struvite stones
About 10–15% of urinary calculi are composed of struvite (ammonium magnesium phosphate, $NH_4MgPO_4 \cdot 6H_2O$).[112] Struvite stones (also known as "infection stones", urease or triple-phosphate stones), form most often in the presence of infection by urea-splitting bacteria.. These infection stones are commonly observed in people who have factors that predispose them to urinary tract infections, such as those with spinal cord injury and other forms of neurogenic bladder, ileal conduit urinary diversion, vesicoureteral reflux, and obstructive uropathies. They are also commonly seen in people with underlying metabolic disorders, such as idiopathic hypercalciuria, hyperparathyroidism, and gout. Infection stones can grow rapidly, forming large calyceal staghorn (antler-shaped) calculi requiring invasive surgery such as percutaneous nephrolithotomy for definitive treatment.[112]

Uric acid stones
About 5–10% of all stones are formed from uric acid.[113] People with certain metabolic abnormalities, including obesity,[114] may produce uric acid stones. They also may form in association with conditions that cause hyperuricosuria (an excessive amount of uric acid in the urine) with or without hyperuricemia (an excessive amount of uric acid in the serum).

Other types
Urolithiasis has also been noted to occur in the setting of therapeutic drug use, with crystals of drug forming within the renal tract in some people currently being treated with agents such as indinavir,[115] sulfadiazine[116] and triamterene.[117]

24. URINARY TRACT INFECTION

"Tell us please, what treatment in an emergency is administered by ear?"....I met his gaze and I did not blink. "Words of comfort," I said to my father." Unknown

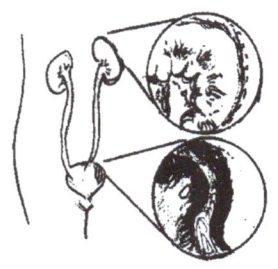

INFLAMMATION IN KIDNEY & URINARY BLADDER

HOW TO IDENTIFY IT?
1. Pain while passing urine and also strong urge to urinate even after bladder is emptied.
2. Pain in the abdominal area and at times radiating to the back.
3. Passing high coloured urine at times
4. Fever with chills and rigors.
5. Nausea and vomiting may be present at times

HOW TO DEAL?
- **STEP 1** If one has the above signs and symptoms, consultation is important in order to prevent further complications as the severity of Urinary tract Infection has to be determined.
- **STEP 2** The antibiotics as prescribed has to be completed in the stipulated dosage and timings in order to prevent recurrence.
- **STEP 3** Proper water intake, personal hygiene and follow up are all equally important to avoid complications.

WHAT WILL BE DONE IN THE HOSPITAL?
A complete physical examination will be done and a urine sample will be collected to look for white blood cells, red blood cells, bacteria, and to test for certain chemicals, such as nitrites. This will be done immediately depending on the condition.

Urine culture will be requested to identify the bacteria and its sensitivity to different type of antibiotics will be known and the best antibiotic will be given.

Complete Blood Count and a blood culture will be done if necessary.

If the infection is severe and person has associated fever, this will be treated aggressively with intravenous antibiotics and other symptomatic measures.

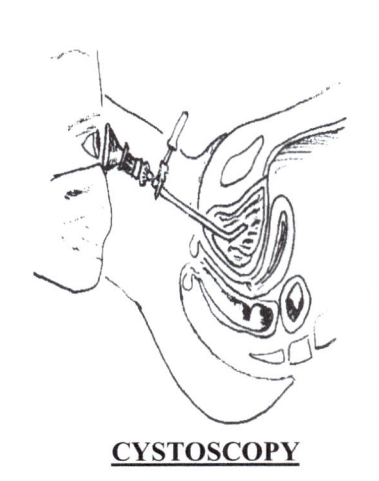
CYSTOSCOPY

Care will be taken to see that there is adequate hydration and further investigations will be requested to know the extent of infection. This will include CT of the abdomen, intravenous pyelogram, ultrasound and voiding cystourethrogram.
For moderate urinary tract infections one will be given antibiotics for 7 days and observed. Commonly used antibiotics include trimethoprim-sulfamethaxozole, Amoxicillin, Augmentin,, doxycycline and fluroquinolones.
In mild cases antibiotics used as mentioned above will show sufficient response

IMPORTANT AND ADVANCED INFORMATION
COMMON CAUSES
E. coli is the cause of 80–85% of urinary tract infections, with *Staphylococcus saprophyticus* being the cause in 5–10%.[118] Rarely they may be due to viral or fungal infections.[119] Other bacterial causes include: *Klebsiella*, *Proteus*, *Pseudomonas*, and *Enterobacter*. Urinary tract infections due to *Staphylococcus aureus* typically occur secondary to blood-borne infections.[120]

Sex
In young sexually active women, sexual activity is the cause of 75–90% of bladder infections, with the risk of infection related to the frequency of sex.[118] The term "honeymoon cystitis" has been applied to this phenomenon of frequent UTIs during early marriage. In post-menopausal women, sexual activity does not affect the risk of developing a UTI. Spermicide use, independent of sexual frequency, increases the risk of UTIs.[118]
Women are more prone to UTIs than men because, in females, the urethra is much shorter and closer to the anus.[121] Urinary catheters
Urinary catheterization increases the risk for urinary tract infections. The risk of bacteriuria (bacteria in the urine) is between 3-6% per day and prophylactic antibiotics are not effective in decreasing symptomatic infections.[121]

Others
A predisposition for bladder infections may run in families. Other risk factors include diabetes,[118] being uncircumcised, and having a large prostate.[120] Complicating factors are rather vague and include predisposing anatomic, functional, or metabolic abnormalities.[122] In children UTIs are associated with vesicoureteral reflux (an abnormal movement of urine from the bladder into ureters or kidneys) and constipation.[123]
Persons with spinal cord injury are at increased risk for urinary tract infection in part because of chronic use of catheter, and in part because of voiding dysfunction.[124]

25. ACUTE RETENTION OF URINE

"There is no medicine like hope, no incentive so great, and no tonic so powerful as expectation of something better tomorrow" Arabic proverb

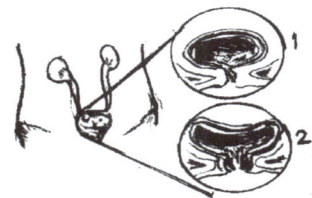

RETENTION OF URINE
1.NORMAL   2.UNDER PRESURRE

HOW TO IDENTIFY IT?
1. Difficulty in passing urine.
2. Distension of the lower part of abdomen.
3. Pain abdomen.
4. There may be dribbling of urine.
5. At times there will be history of past catheterization.

HOW TO DEAL?
- STEP 1 Initially one can try to put effort by trying to force urination in front of running water.
- STEP 2 If not successful, proceed to EMERGENCY DEPARTMENT for need of further assessment and management.
- STEP 3 In many cases where there is past history of retention of urine and has been catheterized, will need recatheterization which at times is done by Paramedic staff at home.
- STEP 4 Never forcefully put a a catheter as this may cause trauma to the ureter.

WHAT WILL BE DONE IN THE HOSPITAL?
A physical examination will usually be done.
If one cannot urinate catheterization will be done after explanation. Taking aseptic measures and after proper lubrication of a Foley's catheter, the tube will be passed up the penis into the bladder and urine is drained. Half of these men will be able to urinate again after catheterization. Depending on the situation the tube will be left insitu or removed later.
Those who do not improve will need surgery if necessary depending upon the condition. This will be necessary if one has partial blockage in the urethra that is causing repeated urinary tract infections, bladder stones, or bladder damage.
Transurethral resection of the prostate (TURP) will be the surgery for benign prostatic hyperplasia which is most commonly used in which a part of the prostate will be removed.

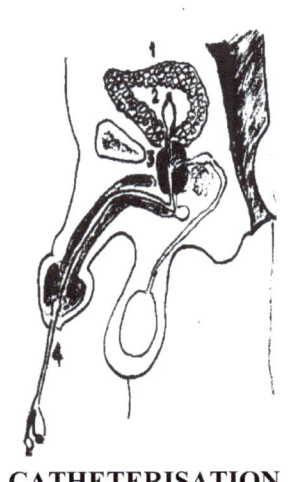
CATHETERISATION

IMPORTANT AND ADVANCED INFORMATION
COMMON CAUSES
In the bladder
Detrusor sphincter dyssynergia
Neurogenic bladder (commonly pelvic splanchic nerve damage, cauda equina syndrome, descending cortical fibers lesion, pontine micturation or storage center lesions, demyelinating diseases or Parkinson's disease)
Iatrogenic (caused by medical treatment/procedure) scarring of the bladder neck (commonly from removal of indwelling catheters or cystoscopy operations)[108]

Damage to the bladder
In the prostate
Benign prostatic hyperplasia (BPH)
Prostate cancer and other pelvic malignancies
Prostatitis
Penile urethra
Congenital urethral valves
Phimosis or pinhole meatus
Circumcision
Obstruction in the urethra, for example a metastasis or a precipitated pseudogout crystal in the urine
STD lesions (gonorrhoea causes numerous strictures, leading to a "rosary bead" appearance, whereas chlamydia usually causes a single stricture)
Other
Tethered spinal cord syndrome
Paruresis ("shy bladder syndrome")- in extreme cases, urinary retention can result
Consumption of some psychoactive substances, mainly stimulants, such as MDMA and amphetamine.
Use of NSAIDs or drugs with anticholinergic properties.
Stones or metastases can theoretically appear anywhere along the urinary tract, but vary in frequency depending on anatomy
Muscarinic antagonist such as Atropine and Scopolamine
Paruresis, inability to urinate in the presence of others (such as in a public restroom), may also be classified as a type of urinary retention, although it is psychological rather than biological.
Brain Mental retardation[108]

26. RENAL FAILURE

"The purpose of medicine is to prevent significant disease, to decrease pain and to postpone death... Technology has to support these goals-if not, it may even be counterproductive." - Medscape

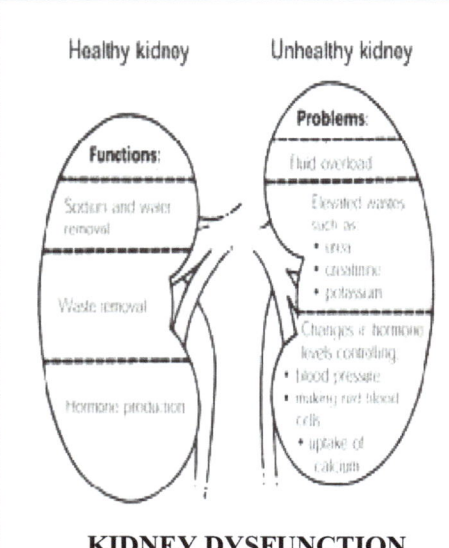

KIDNEY DYSFUNCTION

HOW TO IDENTIFY IT?
1. Less amount of urination.
2. Swelling of lower limbs.
3. At times generalized swelling and puffiness of face.
4. Persisitent weakness with body pain and malaise.
5. Discoloration of the skin.

HOW TO DEAL?
- **STEP 1** Proceed to EMEGENCY DEPARTMENT if one expects Renal Failure as correct measures are very important in order to avoid later complications.
- **STEP 2** Once diagnosed as Renal Failure depending on the status of kidney, person may be subjected to initial medications with frequent follow up or will be put on dialysis which has to be strictly adhered to.
- **STEP 3** If person has to be managed by dialysis it will be either by Hemodialysis or Peritoneal dialysis. Peritoneal dialysis can be done at home using aseptic conditions and under proper supervision.
- **STEP 4** Following a special diet and instructions as specified by the proper authority to maintain normal levels of body electrolytes must be implemented.
- **STEP 5** Fluid overload must be avoided at all costs.

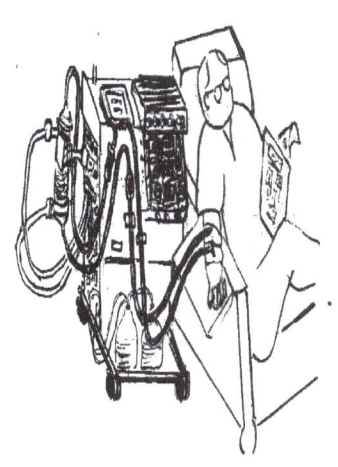
HEMODIALYSIS

WHAT WILL BE DONE IN THE HOSPITAL?
If renal failure has occurred due to severe dehydration or shock this will be corrected initially as in management of SHOCK on page 9.

If symptoms of renal failure develop, initially all relevant blood and urine will be asked. Blood investigations will be of renal profile and all electrolytes.

Ultrasound and other imaging studies will also help to detect any abnormality.

If any medications given is causing the problem to the kidney, an alternative medication will be recommended

If there is blockage in the urinary tract, this will be rectified.

Ultimately dialysis will be considered if wastes are building up in the body as these have to be removed as early as possible.

Dialysis will be either Hemodialysis wherein a machine does the work of the kidneys until they recover or a peritoneal dialysis which can be done at home under proper supervision.

Anemia will be treated with transfusions if it is severe.

Cardiac symptoms will be treated with ACE inhibitor at low doses. To reduce fluid retention diuretics will be prescribed. Multivitamins will be recommended.

Presently a kidney transplant advise will be also suggested and done where possible as this is more beneficial in the long run.

IMPORTANT AND ADVANCED INFORMATION
COMMON CAUSES
Prerenal These include systemic causes, such as low blood volume, low blood pressure, heart failure, and local changes to the blood vessels supplying the kidney.

Intrinsic Common causes are glomerulonephritis, acute tubular necrosis (ATN), and acute interstitial nephritis (AIN).

Postrenal This may be related to benign prostatic hyperplasia, kidney stones, obstructed urinary catheter, bladder stone, bladder, ureteral or renal malignancy.[108]

27. ARTHRITIS

"Lost wealth may be replaced by industry, lost knowledge by study, lost health by temperance or medicine; but lost time is gone forever" Samuel Smiles

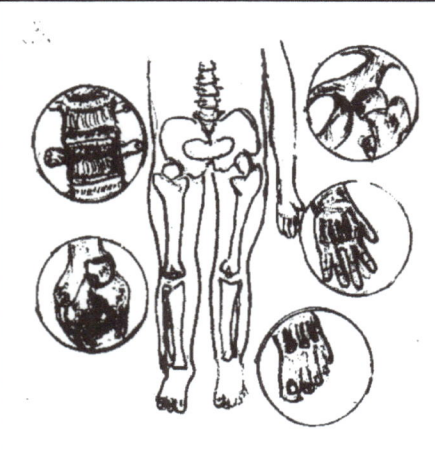

MULTIPLE JOINTS INVOLVED

HOW TO IDENTIFY IT?
1. Swelling of the joints.
2. Pain in the joints.
3. Redness of the joints.
4. Stiffness and unable to move and bend the joints.
5. Pain in the joints at times will be related with diet especially consumption of red meat and less water.

HOW TO DEAL?
- **STEP 1 if swelling of the joints has occurred due to trauma, one will have to see in the EMERGENCY DEPARTMENT for need of further assessment and management.**
- **STEP 2 Cause of the first time swelling of the joint has to be ascertained and if this causes considerable redness or is painful one may need to be evaluated further.**
- **STEP3 In case of arthritis due to known cause, one can initially use dry heat from a heating pad or moist heat in the form of a hot water bottle wrapped in a towel to help relieve pain and stiffness.**
- **STEP 4 Medications to decrease pain like Acetaminophen or Ibuprofen along with local application of anti-inflammatory creams belonging to non steroidal group will also help.**
- **STEP 5 Mobility of the joints is equally important and exercises as recommended by a physiotherapist will help to avoid later difficulties.**

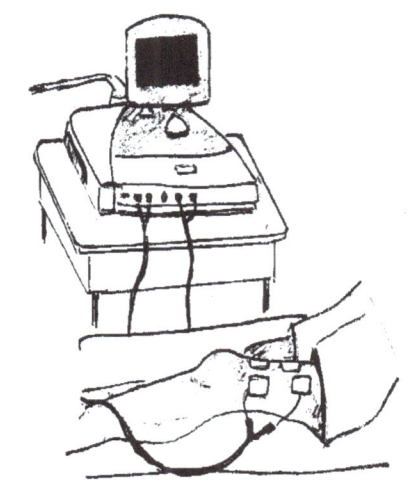

PHYSIOTHERAPY IS IMPORTANT

WHAT WILL BE DONE IN THE HOSPITAL?

Initially a thorough examination of he joint will be made to ascertain cause of the joint swelling or pain. If in considerable pain, analgesics like Brufen or Acetaminophen will be given.

If considerable swelling is there, fluid will be removed from the joint with a needle and this will be sent for further investigations if necessary to rule out infection and other causes like gout

X-rays will also be requested and person with arthritis will be further evaluated by an Orthopedician.

Persons with arthritis will also need long term strategic plans with care from a physiotherapist who will recommend Infrared red ray therapy, proper mobilization exercises and other guide lines for every day activities.

IMPORTANT AND ADVANCED INFORMATION
COMMON CAUSES

There are several diseases where joint pain is primary, and is considered the main feature. Generally when a person has "arthritis" it means that they have one of these diseases, which include:

Osteoarthritis
Rheumatoid arthritis
Gout and pseudo-gout
Septic arthritis
Ankylosing spondylitis
Juvenile idiopathic arthritis
Still's disease

Joint pain can also be a symptom of other diseases. In this case, the arthritis is considered to be secondary to the main disease; these include:
Psoriasis (Psoriatic arthritis), Reactive arthritis, Ehlers-Danlos Syndrome, Haemochromatosis, Hepatitis, Lyme disease, Henoch-Schönlein purpura, Inflammatory bowel disease (Including Crohn's Disease and Ulcerative Colitis), Hyperimmunoglobulinemia D with recurrent fever, Sarcoidosis,
TNF receptor associated periodic syndrome, Wegener's granulomatosis (and many other vasculitis syndromes), Familial Mediterranean fever
Systemic lupus erythematosus[108]

28. NEAR DROWNING

"Drowning... A death in which one is completely overcome by a natural force too great for one to fight.." - Medscape

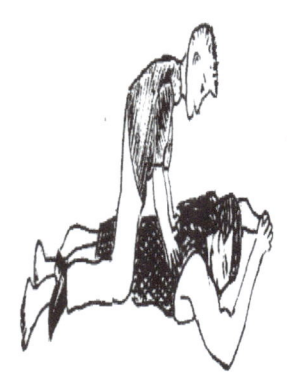

RESUCSITATION IN NEAR DROWNING

HOW TO IDENTIFY IT?
1. After being submerged in water there may be bluish discoloration of face and the body.
2. Frothing from the mouth may be present.
3. There may be less respiratory efforts or absence of breathing.
4. The person may be unconscious.
5. Abdominal distension may be present.

HOW TO DEAL?
- **STEP 1** Call for EMERGENCY ASSISTANCE immediately
- **STEP 2** Depending on the status and if person is not breathing start CPR as on page 118. Since chest compressions are ineffective in water the person must be removed from water
- **STEP 3** Rescue breathing will have to be done till person is removed from water
- **STEP 4** If a floatable immobilization device such as a spine board is available, it should be placed under the person.
- **STEP 5** Stabilization of the neck in all cases must be remembered in case of suspected neck injury.

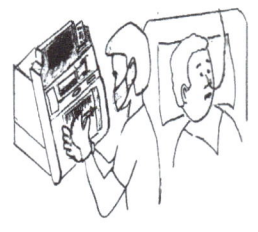

ACID BASE IMBALANCE ESTIMATION IN NEAR DROWNING

WHAT IS DONE IN A HOSPITAL?

After a quick complete assessment, depending on the condition of the person , resuscitative measures will be continued and advanced measures will be initiated in the hospital.. This will mainly involve giving high supplemented level of oxygen and person will be put on a mechanical support by means of a ventilator. Sodium bicarbonate to restore the acid base level to normal values will be given.

Subsequently the blood gases will be monitored to determine how long to continue administering bicarbonate (being given by IV) and ventilatory support

High supplemental levels of oxygen inhalation will be continued until the arterial blood-gas studies show that lower oxygen concentrations are required. When the oxygen in the arteries and the acid-base levels improve, the person will usually regains consciousness.

Other measures will include giving bronchodilators (medications to open up the airway passages) either by nebulization or through a vein.

A chest x-ray will be taken to check for pneumonia or pulmonary edema (congestion of the pulmonary air spaces) and antibiotics will be given to combat any pneumonitis .

All persons with near drowning will be observed and discharged only when proved that the person is safe.

IMPORTANT AND ADVANCED INFORMATION
COMMON CAUSES

Approximately 90% of drownings take place in freshwater (rivers, lakes and swimming pools) and 10% in seawater. Drownings in other fluids is rare, and often relates to industrial accidents.

People have drowned in as little as 30 mm of water lying face down.

Children have drowned in baths, buckets and toilets; inebriates or those under the influence of drugs have died in puddles.

Secondary drowning - Inhaled fluid can act as an irritant inside the lungs. Physiological responses to even small quantities include the extrusion of liquid into the lungs (pulmonary edema) over the following hours, but this reduces the ability to exchange air and can lead to a person "drowning in their own body fluid". Certain poisonous vapors or gases (as for example in chemical warfare), or vomit can have a similar effect. The reaction can take place up to 72 hours after a near drowning incident, and may lead to a serious condition or death. [108]

29. ELECTRICAL INJURIES

"Electricity is actually made up of extremely tiny particles called electrons that one cannot see with the naked eye unless one has been drinking." - Unknown

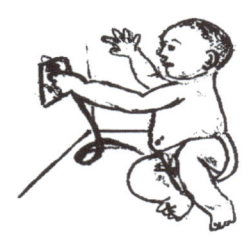

AWARENESS ABOUT ELECRTICITY & CHILDREN

HOW TO IDENTIFY IT?
1. History of exposure to shock from electrical devices.
2. There may be altered level of consciousness.
3. At times numbness of face, arms or legs may be present.
4. Irregularity in pulse.
5. In severe cases burns may be present.

HOW TO DEAL?
- **STEP 1** Always make sure that one is safe before proceeding to the next step in order to avoid injury to oneself.
- **STEP 2** Shut off the electrical current first by unplugging the cord or by removing the fuse.
- **STEP 3** Call for EMERGENCY help.
- **STEP 4** Use a nonconducting object such as a broom or a chair to push the victim from the source of current.
- **STEP 5** When one is sure that the victim is free from electricity, examine the person and start CPR (see page 118) if there is no breathing or pulse.
- **STEP 6** When burns are present, these have to be taken care of (see page 88).
- **STEP 7** If in shock stage handle as given in Shock (see page 8).
- **STEP 8** Traumatic injuries have to be handled also where necessary.

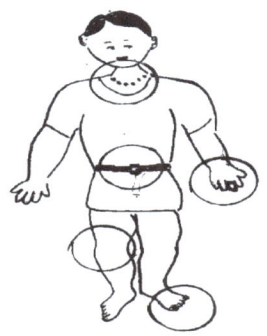

POINT OF ENTRY FROM NECKLACE, BELT & RING
POINT OF EXIT FROM KNEE AND FOOT

WHAT WILL BE DONE IN THE HOSPITAL?

A complete examination will be made and if person is in shock stage, will be handled as per SHOCK on page 9. Treatment will depend on the extent of injuries detected and will be treated accordingly.

In addition Electrocardiogram will be done along with blood investigations to detect any abnormality. At times imaging studies such as CT scan or Magnetic Resonance Imaging will be considered when internal injuries are suspected.

IMPORTANT AND ADVANCED INFORMATION
COMMON CAUSES

Electrical burns can be caused by a variety of ways such as touching or grasping electrically live objects, short-circuiting, inserting fingers into electrical sockets, and falling into electrified water. Lightning strikes are also a cause of electrical burns, but this is a less common event.[125] With the advances in technology, electrical injuries are becoming more common and are the fourth leading cause of work-related traumatic death.[126] One third of all electrical traumas and most high-voltage injuries are job related, and more than 50% of these injures result from power line contact.[126]

Electrical burns can be classified into six categories:

Low-voltage burn. A burn produced by contact with a power source of 500 volts or less is classified as a low-voltage burn. This type of burn may be mild, superficial, or severe depending on the contact time.[127]

High voltage burn. This burn is very severe as the victim makes direct contact with the high voltage supply and the damage runs its course throughout the body. In this case, subdermal tissues are severely damaged.[128]

Arc burn. This type of burn occurs when electrical energy passes from a high-resistance area to a low-resistance area.[129] No contact is required with an arc burn as the electricity ionizes air particles to complete the circuit**Flash burn**. Flash burns are caused by electrical arcs that pass over the skin. . Although the burns on the skin are largely superficial and cover a large area, tissues beneath the skin are generally undamaged and unaffected.[129]

Flame burn. Associated with flash and arc burns, flame burns are caused by contact to objects that were ignited by an electrical source.[129]

Oral burns. This is caused by biting or sucking on electrical cords, and it most commonly happens to children.[130] Electrical current typically passes from one side of the child's mouth to the other, possibly causing deformity.

30. HEAT ILLNESS

"If you're thirsty, you're already about a liter low." Medscape

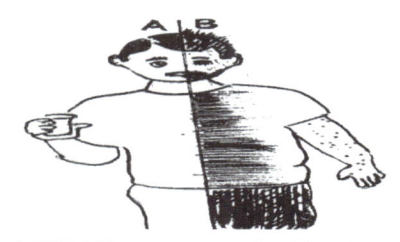

A. **HEAT EXHAUSTION**
MOIST CLAMMY SKIN
NORMAL OR SUB NORMAL TEMP.

B. **HEAT STROKE**
DRY, HOT SKIN
VERY HIGH BODY TEMP.

HOW TO IDENTIFY IT?

HEAT EXHAUSTION
1. Feeling weak.
2. Profuse sweating
3. Thirsty and passing dark coloured urine.
4. At times nausea and vomiting.
5. Dizziness or giddiness

HEAT STROKE
1. Altered behavior initially later can become unconscious
2. At times appears in comatose state.
3. Skin becomes very dry.
4. Respiration becomes irregular.
5. Pulse may be weak.

HOW TO DEAL?

- STEP 1 Awareness is important. Always check for insidious signs when exposed to a hot atmosphere.
- STEP 2 If person has evidence of heat stroke proceed to the EMERGENCY DEPARTMENT immediately as this will need intensive care.
- STEP 3 If in case of Shock stage follow steps as on page 8.
- STEP 4 In case of heat exhaustion oral rehydration has to be commenced by giving prepacked fluids where available every quarter hourly as tolerated. A salted solution can be prepared by adding a teaspoon of salt to a quart (150 ml) of water.
- STEP5 Apply wet cloths to the person's skin and use a fan to lower the body temperature preferably underneath the person's neck, groins and arm pits.
- STEP 6 For muscular cramps, massage gently, but firmly over the affected muscles after giving oral fluids.

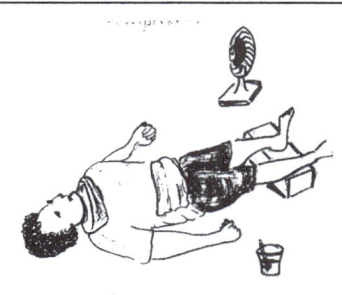

**HAVE PERSON LIE DOWN
APPLY COLD COMPRESS
FAN TO LOWER TEMPER-
ATURE
GIVE FLUIDS**

WHAT WILL BE DONE IN THE HOSPITAL?

Emergency measures will be taken when person is in a Heat Stroke stage. Continuous monitoring will be carried out and if in shock will be treated as in SHOCK on page 9.

Core body temperature reduction will be attempted by applying warm water mist over the body or with towels soaked in warm water and put over the body surface. Fanning will also be done to be directed by continuous airflow over the moistened skin surface.

Body electrolytes will be checked regularly and treated accordingly. Heat exhaustion will need observation of symptoms such as muscle cramps and thirst. Oral rehydration will always be initiated first and observed subsequently.

IMPORTANT AND ADVANCED INFORMATION
COMMON CAUSES.

Heat stroke occurs when thermoregulation is overwhelmed by a combination of excessive metabolic production of heat (exertion), excessive environmental heat, and insufficient or impaired heat loss, resulting in an abnormally high body temperature.[131] In severe cases, temperatures can exceed 40 °C (104 °F).[132] Heat stroke may be *non-exertional* (classic) or *exertional*.

Drugs Some drugs cause excessive internal heat production.[131] The rate of drug-induced hyperthermia is higher where use of these drugs is higher.[131] Many psychotropic medications, such as selective serotonin reuptake inhibitors (SSRIs), monoamine oxidase inhibitors (MAOIs), and tricyclic antidepressants, can cause hyperthermia.[131]

Malignant hyperthermia is a rare reaction to common anesthetic agents (such as halothane) or the paralytic agent succinylcholine. Those who suffer this reaction, which is potentially fatal, have a genetic predisposition.[131]

Personal protective equipment Those working in industry, the military and first responders,[133] may be required to wear Personal Protective Equipment (PPE) against hazards such as chemical agents, gases, fire, small arms and even Improvised Explosive Devices (IEDs). PPE includes a range of hazmat suits, firefighting turnout gear, body armor and bomb suits, amongst others.

Other rare causes of hyperthermia include thyrotoxicosis and an adrenal gland tumor, called pheochromocytoma, both of which can cause increased heat production.[131] Damage to the central nervous system, from brain hemorrhage, status epilepticus, and other kinds of injury to the hypothalamus can also cause hyperthermia.[131]

31. ALCOHOL INTOXICATION

"Alcohol is barren. The words a man speaks in the night of drunkenness fade like the darkness itself at the coming of day." AAA

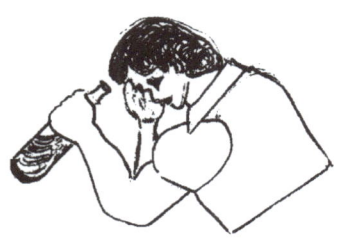

EXCESS ALCOHOL CAUSES INTOXICATION

HOW TO IDENTIFY IT?
1. Smells of alcohol consumption.
2. Abnormal behavior.
3. At times vomiting with pain abdomen.
4. Seizures.
5. Unconsciousness.

HOW TO DEAL?
- STEP 1 Identification about the extent of alcohol intoxication is important.
- STEP 2 If person is in a state of Shock, manage as per on Shock on page 8.
- STEP 3 Handling the person at times involve keeping the person safe and to prevent the person from driving, active physical activities like cycling, swimming, skating and like.
- STEP 4 Keep the person away from machinery.

WHAT WILL BE DONE IN THE HOSPITAL?
In case of confirmed severe alcohol intoxication a gastric lavage will be done if less than one hour has passed.

Further treatment will depend on the state of alcohol intoxication and arterial blood gas, urea and electrolyte and blood glucose level along with alcohol level will be requested and corrected respectively.

At times hemodialysis will be considered if person does not show good response to initial management.

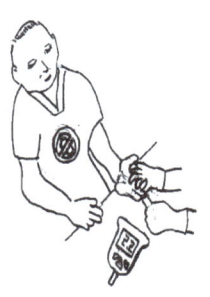

CHECK GLUCOSE VALUE ALWAYS IN ALCOHOLISM

Nausea, vomiting and associated gastritis will be corrected with parenteral medications and intravenous fluids.

Assessment for low blood glucose level will be carried out frequently and corrected.

When there is associated hallucinations, benzodiazepes will be used to lessen and also to lessen the tension and to slow down the symptoms of central nervous system.

Persons going through mild to moderate symptoms will be monitored to make sure that more severe symptoms do not develop.

IMPORTANT AND ADVANCED INFORMATION
DRUG THERAPY

Acamprosate (Campral) stabilises the brain chemistry that is altered due to alcohol dependence via antagonising the actions of glutamate, a neurotransmitter which is hyperactive in the post-withdrawal phase.[134]

Baclofen is an agonist for the GABAB receptors[135][136] which suppresses the motivation to consume cocaine, heroin, alcohol, nicotine and d-amphetamine [137] by inhibiting both withdrawal symptoms and cravings.[138]

Benzodiazepines, while useful in the management of acute alcohol withdrawal, if used long-term can cause a worse outcome in alcoholism. This class of drugs is commonly prescribed to alcoholics for insomnia or anxiety management.[139]

Calcium carbimide (Temposil) works in the same way as disulfiram; it has an advantage in that the occasional adverse effects of disulfiram, hepatotoxicity and drowsiness, do not occur with calcium carbimide.[140][141]

Disulfiram (Antabuse) prevents the elimination of acetaldehyde, a chemical the body produces when breaking down ethanol. The overall effect is severe discomfort when alcohol is ingested: an extremely fast-acting and long-lasting uncomfortable hangover. This discourages an alcoholic from drinking in significant amounts while they take the medicine.

Naltrexone is a competitive antagonist for opioid receptors, effectively blocking the effects of endorphins and opiates. Naltrexone is used to decrease cravings for alcohol and encourage abstinence.

The **CAGE questionnaire,** named for its four questions, is one such example that may be used to screen patients quickly in a doctor's office.

Two "yes" responses indicate that the respondent should be investigated further. The questionnaire asks the following questions:

1. Have you ever felt you needed to **C**ut down on your drinking?
2. Have people **A**nnoyed you by criticizing your drinking?
3. Have you ever felt **G**uilty about drinking?
4. Have you ever felt you needed a drink first thing in the morning (**E**ye-opener) to steady your nerves or to get rid of a hangover?[142][143]

32. SEIZURES IN CHILDREN

"Nobody realizes that some individuals expend tremendous energy merely to be normal." ~Albert Camus

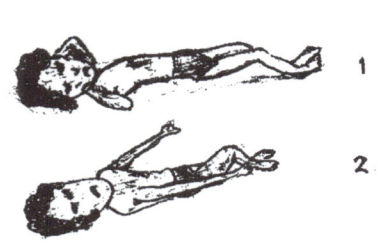

SEIZURES IN CHILDREN
1. TONIC PHASE
2. CLONIC PHASE

HOW TO IDENTIFY IT?
1. Sudden twitching of the body.
2. Loss of consciousness.
3. Frothing from mouth.
4. Body at times can become bluish.
5. There may be clonic movements at times.

HOW TO DEAL?
- **STEP 1** Make sure that airway is patent in every fitting child. Loosen tight clothings around the head or neck. Do not put anything in the mouth.
- **STEP 2** If the child is vomiting, roll the child on to the side and clear out the mouth.
- **STEP 3** In case of associated high temperature and if there has been a past history of similar episode this can be considered as Febrile Convulsions and rectal Diazepam as supplied earlier in the proper dosage can be given. Sponging of the child with warm water to bring down the temperature must be done.
  Do not use ice or cold water as this can cause shivering.
- **STEP 3** Constant observation is very important and if this has been the first seizure attack, proceed to the EMERGENCY DEPARTMENT for further management.
- **STEP 4** In case of already diagnosed seizure disorder, guidelines as specified earlier by the Doctor must be followed.
- **STEP 5** A child who has a longer seizure than usual or with repeated attacks or never regains consciousness or develop new neurological symptoms must be considered as an EMERGENCY situation and hence seen as early as possible.

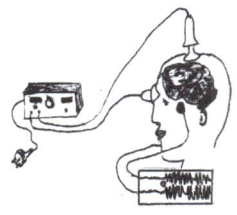

ELECTROENCEHALOGRAM FOR CONFIRMATION

WHAT WILL BE DONE IN THE HOSPITAL?

If a child has seizures which is not initially controlled by medications and is continuous, this will be considered as Status Epilepticus and will have to be treated very aggressively. At times this will need repeated doses of anti seizure medication along with continuous monitoring. Anesthetist consultation will be considered and if necessary mechanical ventilation will be done under deep sedation.

In other cases , initially it will be necessary to rule out other conditions such as non epileptic seizures. All seizures will be managed with oxygen care, airway maintenance and intravenous or rectal diazepam.
Blood glucose will be checked and corrected if necessary.
If temperature is more than 38 degree C will be treated with rectal paracetamol. Also a thorough check will be made to find any source of infection especially meningitis and necessary investigations will be carried out.
If the cause of seizures is not from infection an Electroencephalogram will be considered necessary and further treatment will be based on that..

IMPORTANT AND ADVANCED INFORMATION
COMMON CAUSES
This classification is based on observation (clinical and EEG)
I Partial seizures
A Simple partial seizures - consciousness is not impaired
1 With motor signs **2** With sensory symptoms **3** With autonomic symptoms or signs **4** With psychic symptoms
B Complex partial seizures - consciousness is impaired
1 Simple partial onset, followed by impairment of consciousness
2 With impairment of consciousness at onset
C Partial seizures evolving to secondarily generalized seizures
1 Simple partial seizures evolving to generalized seizures
2 Complex partial seizures evolving to generalized seizures
3 Simple partial seizures evolving to complex partial seizures evolving to generalized seizures
II Generalized seizures
A Absence seizures
1 Typical absence seizures **2** Atypical absence seizures
B Myoclonic seizures
C Clonic seizures **D** Tonic seizures **E** Tonic–clonic seizures **F** Atonic seizures
III Unclassified epileptic seizures[108]

33. POISONS

> "All substances are poisonous, there is none that is not a poison; the right dose differentiates a poison from a remedy." -Medscape

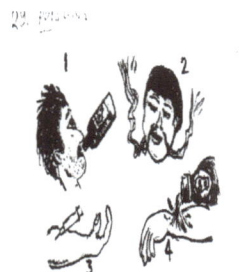

POISONS
1. SWALLOWED
2. INHALED
3. INJECTED
4. ABSORBED

HOW TO IDENTIFY IT?
1. Presence of poisonous substance and history of consumption.
2. At times extremely emotional upset.
3. Vomiting at times and poison related symptoms like smell in case of hydrocarbon substance ingestion.
4. Past history of some ailments.
5. At times deeply unconscious.

HOW TO DEAL?
- **STEP 1** If the poison has been identified and is potentially dangerous, proceed to the nearest EMERGENCY DEPARTMENT taking the responsible substance.
- **STEP 2** If the person is in a comatose stage, handle as per on page 10.
- **STEP 3** If poison has spilt over the skin or gone into the eye wash thoroughly with clean water before proceeding.
- **STEP 4** Gravity of situation cannot be underestimated and all poisonous substances ingested must be evaluated since delay can be life threatening especially in children.
- **STEP 5** Watchful waiting in a Hospital is better than at home as one can be prepared to treat complications at once.

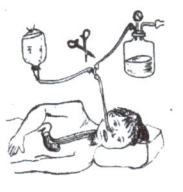

GASTRIC LAVAGE

WHAT WILL BE DONE IN THE HOSPITAL?

A history and physical examination to look for evidence of poisoning will be performed. If breathing appears inadequate ventilation with oxygen using bag and mask will commence Breathing will be monitored and ventilation will be done if necessary. If in shock will be handled as per SHOCK on page 9.

Supportive care will also involve management of low blood pressure, cardiac problems ,convulsions, temperature maintenance and urine retention.
The doctor will order laboratory tests based on the organ systems that can be harmed by the specific drug overdose. Specific drug levels in the blood will also be measured, depending on the drug taken. Drug screening will also be done if necessary.
The stomach will be washed out by gastric lavage (stomach pumping) to mechanically remove unabsorbed drugs from the stomach. during the detoxification process.
Specific antidotes will be administered where the suspected poison cause is known. Further the person will be admitted for observation.

IMPORTANT AND ADVANCED INFORMATION
COMMON DRUGS CAUSING POISONING & THEIR ANTIDOTES[108]

1 Anticholinergics antidote is Cholinergics and vice versa
2 Antipsychotics (such as Haloperidol and Risperidone) antidote is Ropinirole or Bromocryptine
3 Atropine and /or Scopolomine antidote is Physosigmine
4 Benodiazepene an Barbiturate antidote is Flumazenil
5 Beat blockers (propronolol) antidote is Calcium gluconate and or Glucagon
6 Caffeine and other xanthenes antidote is Adenosine and vice versa
7 Calcium Channel blockers antidote is Calcium gluconate
8 Cyanide antidote is amylnitrate, sodium nitrate, sodium thiosulfate
9 Ethylene glycol antidote is Ethanol or fomepizole and thiamine
10 Hydrochloric acid antidote is Calcium gluconate
11 Iron and other heavy metals antidote is Desferoxamine, Deferasirox
12 Isoniazid antidote is Pyridoxine
13 Magnesium antidote is Calcium gluconate
14 Methanol antidote is Ethanol or fompizole and folinic acid
15 Nicotine antidote is Bupropion and other ganglion blockers
16. Opioids antidote is naloxone
17 Organophsphates antidote is Atropine and pralidoxime
18. Paracetamol (acetaminophen) antidote is N acetylcysteine
19 Vitamin K anticoagulants (warfarin) antidote is Vitamin K

34. BITES AND STINGS

"Reality doesn't bite rather our perception of reality bites" -Livingston

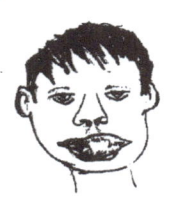

SWELLING OCCURS IN ANY PART OF BODY

HOW TO IDENTIFY IT?

1. History of being bitten.
2. Redness at the site.
3. Swelling at the suspected site.
4. Pain at the site.
5. At times generalized body reaction such as swelling of face and limbs with irregular respiration, altered pulse and person can even become unconscious.

HOW TO DEAL?

- **STEP 1** If a person goes into a Shock after a bite or a sting follow as per on page 8.
- **STEP 2** All bites from animal origin have to be seen and evaluated in an EMERGENCY DEPARTMENT for further care and to prevent complications.
- **STEP 3** At times a person who is exposed to a potentially dangerous situations such as bees when collecting of honey or extraction of venom from snakes must follow the guide lines as specified earlier by the concerned authority.
- **STEP 4** In case of stings, initially pain may be relieved by applying ice pack or one can keep a cool, wet cloth over the surface.
- **STEP 5** Elevate the limb area of the bite or sting to decrease swelling.
- **STEP 6** In adults only, an antihistamine can be given for relief along with a local anesthetic spray where available to decrease pain.
- **STEP 7** Hydrocortisone cream or calamine lotion can be applied locally at the site for relief.

WHAT WILL BE DONE IN THE HOSPITAL?

The person will be examined and the extent of bites and wounds will be recorded. In case of anaphylaxis (shock stage) epinephrine will be immediately given which will reverse the uncomfortable flushing and itching. After getting epinephrine, steroid drugs (such as prednisone or methylprednisolone or hydrocortisone) will be given. Antihistamines will also be given which will help to lessen the itching sensation and also lessen the allergy.

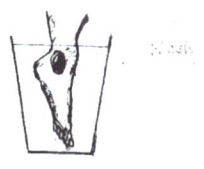

WASH AND SOAK THE AREA

Any person whose tetanus shots are not up-to-date will receive a booster shot. Some wounds will be left open and allowed to heal on their own, while others will require stitches.

Dead and damaged tissue also will be removed.

In cases of suspected rabies, the victim will be given several injections with rabies vaccine over a specific period of time.

Cat bites and human bites, will usually be treated with antibiotics, however antibiotics in other cases will be limited to persons whose injuries or other health problems make them likely candidates for infection.

The person will also require immunization against hepatitis B and other diseases. A follow-up visit will also be requested.

IMPORTANT AND ADVANCED INFORMATION
COMMON CAUSES
Arthropods
Spider bite, Insect bites and stings, Flea bites are responsible for the transmission of bubonic plague, Mosquito bites are responsible for the transmission of dengue fever and malaria.

Vertebrates other than humans
Bites from dogs are commonplace, with children the most common victims and the face the most common target.[144]

Other companion animals, including cats, ferrets, and parrots, may bite humans. Wildlife may sometimes bite humans. The bites of various mammals such as bats, rabbits, wolves, raccoons, etc. may transmit rabies, which is almost always fatal if left untreated.

Involuntary biting injuries due to closed-fist injuries from fists striking teeth (referred to as reverse bite injuries) are a common consequence of fist fights. These have been termed "fight bites". Injuries in which the knuckle joints or tendons of the hand are bitten into tend to be the most serious.

Other
Snakebite, Leech bite

35. ABORTION

"No woman wants an abortion. Either she wants a child or she wishes to avoid pregnancy"-Unknown

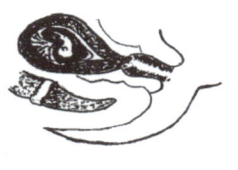

FETUS IN THE WOMB

HOW TO IDENTIFY IT?
PREGNANCY TEST POSITIVE
1. Bleeding heavily from vagina
2. Appears significant pale.
3. At times clotted blood and renants passed out from vagina.
4. If blleding heavy can be in state of shock.
5. Body weakness and giddiness

HOW TO DEAL?
- **STEP 1** If one suspects abortion is likely, or there is moderate to heavy bleeding per vagina in a confirmed early pregnancy state consult a doctor in an EMERGENCY DEPARTMENT as soon as possible.
- **STEP 2** If at times the person is in a state of shock due to heavy bleeding, manage as per page 8.

WHAT WILL BE DONE IN THE HOSPITAL?
Initially if the person is bleeding heavily from the vagina and is in a state of Shock will be handled as in SHOCK on page 9.

All suspected abortion cases will be asked for a urine examination to confirm the pregnancy and a pelvic examination will be done to determine the size and shape of the uterus and also to rule out any ectopic pregnancy. Relevant blood investigations will be asked and an Ultrasound will be done to see the status of the fetus.

If hemoglobin in the blood is significantly low, measures will be taken to increase it by means of a blood transfusion or supplemented iron will be given parenterally or orally.

Person will also be screened for sexual transmitted disease and other type of infections and will be treated.

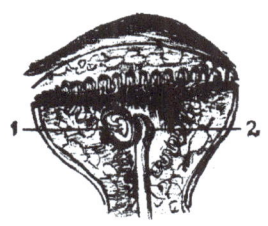

DILATATION AND CURETTAGE
1. FETUS   2. CURETTAGE

If an abortion is inevitable, this will be first confirmed by a specialist. Depending on the weeks of pregnancy further action will include the procedure of dilatation and curettage where the product of conception will be removed under aseptic conditions by experts in their field.

Different procedures will be used for surgical abortion depending on the weeks of pregnancy.

IMPORTANT AND ADVANCED INFORMATION

Practice of Induced Abortion Methods

- MVA
- Dilation and Evacuation
- EVA
- Hysterotomy
- Dilation and Curettage
- Intact D&X
- Mifepristone
- Induced Miscarriage

1st Trimester: 0-12 weeks   2nd Trimester: 12-28 weeks   3rd Trimester: 28-40 weeks

Original uploader was Kaldari at en.wikipedia (reference 108)

36. ECLAMPSIA

"If there's one rule about the type of pregnant woman who develops pre-eclampsia, it's that there are no rules. It's pretty much an equal opportunity disease." - Kathleen Mahoney

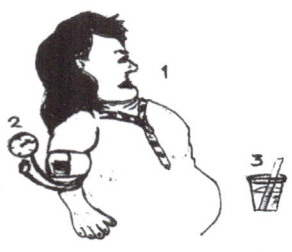

TOXEMIA OF PREGNANCY
1. SWELLING OF FACE/HANDS
2. HIGH BLOOD PRESSURE
3. BLOOD IN URINE

HOW TO IDENTIFY IT?
PREGNANCY TEST POSITIVE
1. Bad headaches.
2. Swelling of lower limbs.
3. Passing high colored urine.
4. Dizziness, unable to walk.
5. At times unconsciousness.

HOW TO DEAL?
- **STEP 1** Frequent vomiting and if blood pressure is found to be in the high range proceed to the EMERGENCY DEPARTMENT for further assessment.
- **STEP 2** If at times the person collapses or goes into a coma follow as per page 10.
- **STAGE 3** One must look out for a swelling of face or limbs and consultation is imminent.
- **STAGE 4** For mild Eclampsia that is not rapidly getting worse, one may have to reduce their level of activity, monitor how they feel and follow up as suggested must be strictly adhered to.

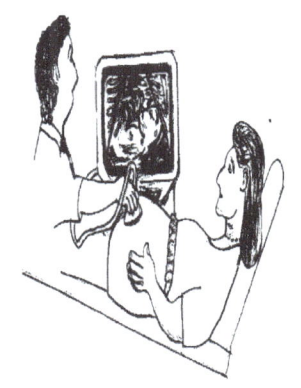

ULTRASOUND TO SEE FETUS IS IMPORTANT

WHAT WILL BE DONE IN THE HOSPITAL?

This depends on the state of presentation. If a pregnant lady develops seizures this will be controlled by anticonvulsants, the drug of choice being Magnesium Sulfate since this is safe both for mother and baby.

In case of severe eclampsia and if in advanced pregnancy state of more than 32 weeks delivery will be the choice in order to avoid complications to both mother and baby.

Blood investigations which will assess the functions of the liver and kidney will be requested and followed up serially.

In stable mild cases pregnancy will be continued up to 36 to 37 weeks.

If less than 34 weeks pregnant and a 24 hour to 48 hour delay is possible with continuous monitoring, antenatal corticosteroids will be given to speed up the fetal lung development before delivery.

IMPORTANT AND ADVANCED INFORMATION
COMMON CAUSES

Eclampsia, like preeclampsia, tends to occur more commonly in first pregnancies and young mothers where it is thought that novel exposure to paternal antigens is involved. Furthermore, women with preexisting vascular diseases (hypertension, diabetes, and nephropathy) or thrombophilic diseases such as the antiphospholipid syndrome are at higher risk to develop preeclampsia and eclampsia. Having a large placenta (multiple gestation, hydatidiform mole) also predisposes women to toxemia. In addition, there is a genetic component: patients whose mother or sister had the condition are at higher risk.[145] Patients who have experienced eclampsia are at increased risk for preeclampsia/eclampsia in a later pregnancy.

37. ECTOPIC PREGNANCY

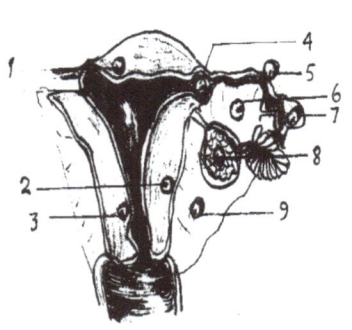

"Each new life, no matter how brief, forever changes the world." Rigveda

DIFFERENT POSITIONS OF THE OVUM
1. INTERSTITIAL 2. INTRAMURAL
3. CERVICAL 4. ISTHMIC TUBAL
5. AMPULLAR TUBAL
6. INTALIGMENTOUS
7. INFUNDIBULAR TUBAL
8. OVARIAN 9. ABDOMINAL

HOW TO IDENTIFY IT?
PREGNANCY TEST POSITIVE
1. Abnormal vaginal bleeding.
2. Pain abdomen usually in the lower part.
3. Persistent vomiting.
4. Bodyache and dizziness.
5. At times loss of consciousness.

HOW TO DEAL?
- STEP 1 If one thinks she is pregnant and has the above symptoms, to see in the EMERGENCY DEPARTMENT.
- STEP 2 Many times one who has an Ectopic Pregnancy will also be in a state of shock in advanced cases. Such cases must be handled as per Shock on page 8.

WHAT WILL BE DONE IN THE HOSPITAL?
Many cases of ectopic pregnancy may present initially in a state of Shock and this will be managed as in SHOCK on page 9.

A thorough physical examination will be done and the size of uterus will be checked and tenderness will be noted and a urine pregnancy test will be done to confirm pregnancy.

Subsequently ultrasound will be done to visualize the position of the fetus and when the position is outside the uterine cavity will be considered an ectopic pregnancy.

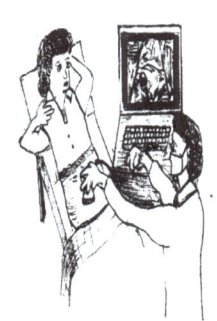

FETUS VISUALIZATION BY ULTRASOUND IS MANDATORY

A confirmed ectopic pregnancy will be considered as an Emergency and treatment will be started immediately to prevent harm to the woman.
Medical line of treatment will be attempted if the pregnancy is found early, and before the fallopian tube has been damaged.
A medication by name Methotrexate will be given which will usually end the pregnancy. This has to be constantly followed up and fore seen for any side effects. If pregnancy has advanced beyond the first few weeks, surgical approach will be done.

Laparoscopic surgery will be feasible where small cuts (incisions) are made over the abdomen and the fetus removed.

IMPORTANT AND ADVANCED INFORMATION

Risk factors include: pelvic inflammatory disease, infertility, use of an intrauterine device (IUD), previous exposure to DES, tubal surgery, intrauterine surgery (e.g. D&C), smoking, previous ectopic pregnancy, and tubal ligation.[146]

Cilial damage and tube occlusion
Women with pelvic inflammatory disease (PID) have a high occurrence of ectopic pregnancy.[147] This results from the build-up of scar tissue in the Fallopian tubes, causing damage to cilia.[148]
Endometrial/pelvic/genital tuberculosis, another cause of Asherman's syndrome, can also lead to ectopic pregnancy as infection may lead to tubal adhesions in addition to intrauterine adhesions.[149]
Tubal ligation can predispose to ectopic pregnancy.
Reversal of tubal sterilization (Tubal reversal) carries a risk for ectopic pregnancy. This is higher if more destructive methods of tubal ligation (tubal cautery, partial removal of the tubes) have been used than less destructive methods (tubal clipping). A history of a tubal pregnancy increases the risk of future occurrences to about 10%.[148] This risk is not reduced by removing the affected tube, even if the other tube appears normal.
Although some investigations have shown that patients may be at higher risk for ectopic pregnancy with advancing age, it is believed that age is a variable which could act as a surrogate for other risk factors. Also, it has been noted that smoking is associated with ectopic risk. Vaginal douching is thought by some to increase ectopic pregnancies.[148]

38. PELVIC INFLAMMATORY DISEASE

"PID can affect the quality of life and also the ability to have children."-Medscape

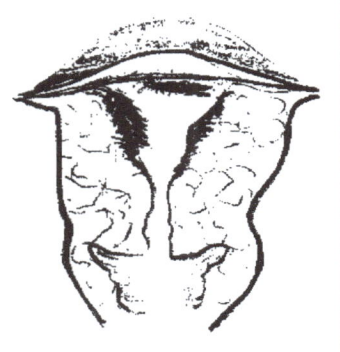

INFLAMMATION AND INFECTION OF THE LINING OF THE UTERUS

HOW TO IDENTIFY IT?
1. Discharge from vagina.
2. Pain abdomen and back pain.
3. Fever may be present.
4. At times urinary disturbance.
5. Feels weak and unable to do normal activity.

HOW TO DEAL?
- **STEP 1** At times when there is high fever with associated vaginal discharge one has to see in an EMERGENCY DEPARTMENT for further evaluation.
- **STEP 2** Persons who are at risk for pelvic inflammatory disease (PID) especially diabetes and immunocompromised people must be evaluated if they have the above mentioned identifiable factors.

WHAT WILL BE DONE IN THE HOSPITAL?
A diagnosis of Pelvic Inflammatory Disease will initially be made after a detailed history taking and an examination. If detected to have associated pregnancy, will be considered on an urgent basis and parenteral antibiotics will be given in a hospital set up initially. If person has not responded to earlier antibiotics and is symptomatic and toxic and there is a possibility of a tuboovarian abscess or localized pus in the uterus surgery will be considered. Diagnostic laparoscopy may be considered at times also.

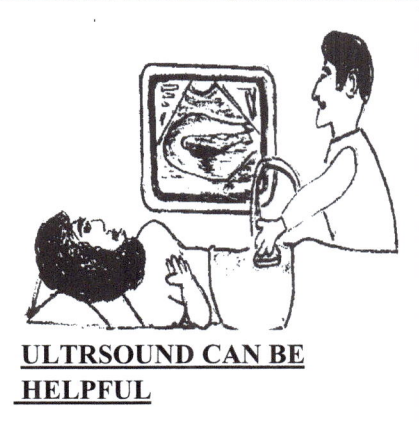
ULTRSOUND CAN BE HELPFUL

All cases of PID will need to have screening for infections and an ultrasound to know the status of the uterus, fallopian tubes or ovaries.

However treatment will be initiated first by proper antibiotics even before awaiting results to give relief and prevent complications depending on the state of PID.

IMPORTANT AND ADVANCED INFORMATION
COMMON CAUSES

Pelvic inflammatory disease (or **disorder**) (**PID**) is a term for inflammation of the uterus, fallopian tubes, and/or ovaries as it progresses to scar formation with adhesions to nearby tissues and organs. This can lead to infertility. PID is a vague term and can refer to viral, fungal, parasitic, though most often bacterial infections. PID should be classified by affected organs, the stage of the infection, and the organism(s) causing it. Although a sexually transmitted infection (STI) is often the cause, many other routes are possible, including lymphatic, postpartum, postabortal (either miscarriage or abortion) or intrauterine device (IUD) related, and hematogenous spread. Two thirds of patients with laparoscopic evidence of previous PID were not aware they had PID.
Complications
PID can cause scarring inside the reproductive organs, which can later cause serious complications, including chronic pelvic pain, infertility, ectopic pregnancy (the leading cause of pregnancy-related deaths in adult females), and other dangerous complications of pregnancy. Occasionally, the infection can spread to in the peritoneum causing inflammation and the formation of scar tissue on the external surface of the liver (Fitz-Hugh-Curtis syndrome). Multiple infections and infections that are treated later are more likely to result in complications.

Fertility may be restored in women affected by PID. Traditionally tuboplastic surgery was the main approach to correct tubal obstruction or adhesion formation, however success rates tended to be very limited. In vitro fertilization (IVF) has been used to bypass tubal problems and has become the main treatment for patients who want to become pregnant.[108]

39. TESTIS TORSION

> "But I hang on to my prejudices, they are the testicles of my mind." Eric Hoffer

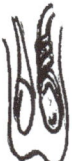

TWISTING OF THE TESTIS

HOW TO IDENTIFY IT?
1. Pain in the scrotum area.
2. Redness at the scrotum site.
3. At times vomiting.
4. Past history of similar episodes but resolved on own.
5. There may be history of injury at times.

HOW TO DEAL?
- **Testicular torsion is an emergency, and the child should be taken to the EMERGENCY DEPARTMENT immediately if he shows the signs or symptoms of testicular torsion.**

WHAT WILL BE DONE IN THE HOSPITAL?

An initial evaluation will be done and seen and seen if the affected testis appear to be higher and for any swelling and discoloration. Further tests will be asked for on an Emergency basis such as Ultrsound scan. Ultrasound scan accompanied by a contrast agent will be more beneficial to know the extent of testicular torsion. Other procedure which is useful is a nuclear scan where a tiny amount of radioactive fluid will be injected into the blood and detected as it flows through the scrotum and testis. If the radioactive fluid does not flow through the testis it is evidential of testicular torsion.

All testicular torsion will be handled on an Emergency basis by a surgeon.

All testicular torsion will be handled on an Emergency basis by a surgeon. Initially the doctor will try to restore blood flow to the testis by hand and to await for subsequent surgery as it is a must since there will be a high possibility of recurrence.

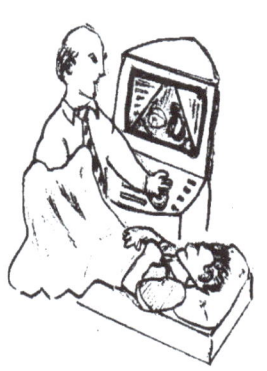
DOPPLER ULTRASOUND IS HELPFUL

Surgical procedure is known as Orchidopexy where the Surgeon makes an incision and will untwist the cord and secure the testis in place so that it will not rotate again. To prevent further testicular torsion, the other testis will also be secured. In radical cases if the testis has not been untwisted in time and has become necrotic (damaged beyond recovery), it will be removed.

IMPORTANT AND ADVANCED INFORMATION
COMMON CAUSES

Congenital
Conditions that allow the testicle to rotate predispose to torsion.[150] A congenital malformation of the processus vaginalis known as the "bell-clapper deformity" accounts for 90% of all cases.[151] In this condition, rather than the testes attaching posteriorly to the inner lining of the scrotum by the mesorchium, the mesorchium terminates early and the testis is free floating in the tunica vaginalis.

Temperature
Torsions are sometimes called "winter syndrome" because they are more frequent in cold conditions, specifically decreasing atmospheric temperature and humidity.[152]

40. ACUTE PSYCHOSIS

"Every normal person, in fact, is only normal on the average. His ego approximates to that of the psychotic in some part or other and to a greater or lesser extent." Sigmund Freud

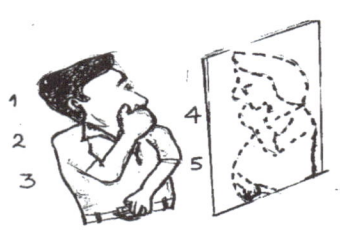

ACUTE PSYCHOSIS
1. DELUSIONS 2. HALLUCINATIONS
3. INCOHERENCE
4. HYPERACTIVITY
5. FLAT AFFECT

HOW TO IDENTIFY IT?
1. Abnormal behavior.
2. Lack of sleep.
3. Confusion.
4. Feels can hear at times unusual sounds, feels something and perceive things that are not there.
5. Not in reality with the world and answers very bizzardly.

HOW TO DEAL?
- **STEP 1** At times the person can be excessively excitable or violent, this will need restraint, always seek assistance first before approaching the person. Seek Ambulance care if necessary.
- **STEP 2** Violent or hysterical persons will also need sedation at times. If past history is present and is being treated, the medication as prescribed earlier have to be given and maintained.
- **STEP 3** At times psychotic patients will go to a hyperventilated state and subsequently can even become comatose, these have to be handled as on page 10.
- **STEP 4** All persons with Psychosis will need utmost attention and have to be constantly observed to prevent self inflicted injuries and also priority about the care taker's safety.

WHAT WILL BE DONE IN THE HOSPITAL?
Initially if the person is found to be excessive excitable, aggressive or violent he or she will be sedated in the Emergency Department. The main drug used will be Haloperidol. Subsequently will be handled by Specialist in the field.

First time diagnosed psychotic persons who are in an unstable state will often be cared for in a hospital to ensure their safety.

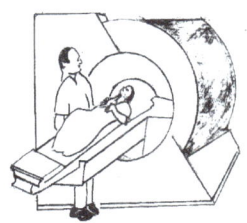

C.T. SCAN (FUNCTIONAL CAUSES MUST ALWAYS BE RULED OUT)

Laboratory and x-ray testing will be done only if necessary to help pinpoint the exact diagnosis. This will involve drug screening and test for syphilis. MRI of the brain will also be requested if necessary to aid in the diagnosis.

The best treatment for bipolar disorder will be a combination of medication and counseling.

Combination of medications and counseling will be carried out. This will often involve treating the maniac symptoms with one group and the depressive symptom with other group. The psychiatric medications which will commonly be used in adults will belong to antidepressants, anxiolytics, antipsychotic and mood stabilizing agents Along with medication, ongoing psychotherapy, or "talk" therapy, will be an important part of treatment for psychiatric conditions. During therapy, one will discuss feelings, thoughts, and behaviors that caused the problems.

Maintenance of steady mood will also be handled by constant elevation and other drugs if necessary.

IMPORTANT AND ADVANCED INFORMATION
COMMON CAUSES

A very large number of medical conditions can cause psychosis, sometimes called *secondary psychosis*.[153] Examples include: disorders causing *delirium* (*toxic psychosis*), in which consciousness is disturbed neurodevelopmental disorders and chromosomal abnormalities, including velocardiofacial syndrome, neurodegenerative disorders, such as Alzheimer's disease,[154] dementia with Lewy bodies,[155] and Parkinson's disease [156], focal neurological disease, such as stroke, brain tumors,[157] multiple sclerosis,[158] and some forms of epilepsy, malignancy (typically via masses in the brain, paraneoplastic syndromes, or drugs used to treat cancer), infectious and postinfectious syndromes, including infections causing delirium, viral encephalitis, HIV,[159] malaria,[160] Lyme disease,[161][162][163] syphilis[164][165], endocrine disease, such as hypothyroidism, hyperthyroidism, adrenal failure, Cushing's syndrome, hypoparathyroidism and hyperparathyroidism; sex hormones also affect psychotic symptoms and sometimes childbirth can provoke psychosis, termed puerperal psychosis, inborn errors of metabolism, such as porphyria and metachromatic leukodystrophy[166][167][168], nutritional deficiency, such as vitamin B_{12} deficiency[169][170]

41. BURNS

"Better do a kindness near at home than go far to burn incense" Chinese proverb

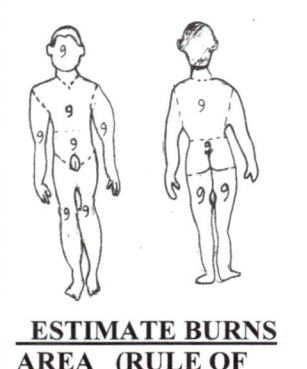

ESTIMATE BURNS AREA (RULE OF NINES IN ADULT)

HOW TO IDENTIFY IT?
1. Redness at site of burns and blisters.
2. Pain depending on the extent of burns.
3. Swelling over the site of burns.
4. Skin becomes charred depending on the type of burns.
5. In case of severe burns, person will be in a state of shock.

HOW TO DEAL?
FOR MAJOR BURNS:
- STEP 1 IF person is on fire, tell the patient to stop, drop and roll. Wrap the person in blanket or thick material to smoothen the flames. Dounce the person with water.
- STEP 2 Make sure that the person is no longer in contact with the source of burns.
- STEP 3 Make sure that the person is breathing. If breathing has stopped or if the person airway is blocked, open the airway. Begin CPR if necessary (See page 118)
- STEP 4 Determine the type and extent of burns, that is the area involved.
- STEP 5 If sustained burns over critical areas such as face, neck or perineum, seek care in the EMERGENCY DEPARTMENT.

FOR MINOR BURNS
- STEP 1 Run cool water over the area of the burn and if the skin is unbroken.
- STEP 2 Later cover the area with a dry, sterile bandage or clean dressing
- STEP 3 Relief of pain can be handled with Actaminophen or Ibuprofen
- STEP 4 Watchful observation is important and seek consultation if there is any signs of infection or is not healing properly or is in considerable pain.

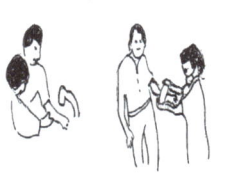

WASH ALWAYS BEFORE FIRST AID

WHAT WILL BE DONE IN THE HOSPITAL?

All burns persons will be assessed initially for the extent of burns using the formula of 9's in adults and the degree of burns. If in shock stage will be handled as in SHOCK on page 9. Severe burns covering large parts of the body will need initially intensive treatment with strong pain killers preferably belonging to the opioid group, intravenous fluids to replace the fluids lost and also the ongoing losses and intravenous antibiotics to prevent infection.

Urine output and other body organ functions will be frequently assessed
Antitetanus injection will be given if not given in the past.
Subsequently third degree burns will also require skin grafts or replacement with synthetic skin.
Second degree burns will also be treated in a Hospital set up in the Burns Unit depending on the extent. Antibiotic cream or other creams or ointments meant for burns will be applied. Fluids assessment will be made and constantly monitored.
First degree burns will be treated with skin care with application of local antibiotics creams and pain relief medications such as Acetaminophen will be given.

IMPORTANT AND ADVANCED INFORMATION
COMMON CAUSES

Thermal Almost half of injuries are due to efforts to fight a fire.[171] Scalding is caused by hot liquids or gases and most commonly occurs from exposure to hot drinks, high temperature tap water in baths or showers, hot cooking oil, or steam.

Chemical Chemical burns can be caused by over 25,000 substances,[172] most of which are either a strong base (55%) or a strong acid (26%).[173] Common agents include: sulfuric acid as found in toilet cleaners, sodium hypochlorite as found in bleach, and halogenated hydrocarbons as found in paint remover, among others.[174]

Electrical The most common causes of electrical burns in children are electrical cords (60%) followed by electrical outlets (14%).[174] Lightning may also result in electrical burns.[175]

Radiation Radiation burns may be caused by protracted exposure to ultraviolet light (such as from the sun, tanning booths or arc welding) or from ionizing radiation (such as from radiation therapy, X-rays or radioactive fallout).[176]

42. HEAD INJURY

"Genuine forgiveness does not deny anger but faces it head-on" Alice Duer Mil-

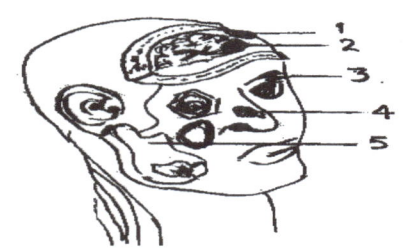

VARIOUS LOCATIONS OF HEAD INJURY 1.EXTRADURAL HEMATOMA 2INTRACRANIAL HEMORRHAGE 3ORBITAL INJURY 4NASOPHARYNGEAL INJURY 5TEMPEROMANDIBULAR

HOW TO IDENTIFY IT?
1. History of trauma with loss of consciousness.
2. At times transcent loss of memory.
3. Presence of swelling over the head may be present at times.
4. Associated headache may be present.
5. At times can be confused and not cooperative.

HOW TO DEAL?

- **CARE DEPENDS UPON THE EXTENT OF INJURY**
  STEP 1 Do a quick assessment and in case if the person is not breathing or there is a deep wound or if in shock, handle as per Shock on page 8. Make sure that there is no neck injury.
- **STEP 2** If one suspects bone injury, proceed to EMERGENCY DEPARTMENT urgently.
- **STEP 3** If bleeding is there from the face, keep the face elevated.
- **STEP 4** If sustained head injury and person is stable, will also need observation and in the event of development of new symptoms, such as vomiting, altered sensorium or difference in the size of pupil, one must see in the EMERGENCY DEPARTMENT.
- **STEP 5** All head injuries are to be considered seriously till proved otherwise.

WHAT WILL BE DONE IN THE HOSPITAL?
All serious head injuries will be managed by a team of specialists depending on the extent and area of involvement.
The doctor will perform a physical exam and may do blood tests, an X-ray, a CT scan, or an EEG depending on the extent of injury such as if there is bleeding from the nose, eyes, or mouth, or nasal blockage ,breaks in the skin (lacerations) or bruising around the eyes or widening of the distance between the eyes, which may mean injury to the bones between the eye sockets.

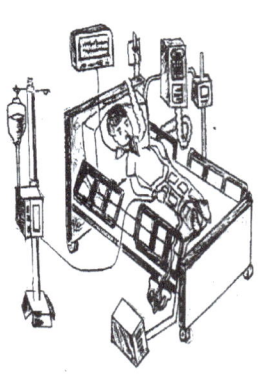
INTENSIVE HEAD INJURY MANAGEMENT

In serious head injury oxygen will be provided and the cervical spine will be protected with importance on airway maintenance and other injuries will be checked
Associated low blood pressure will be corrected by giving intravenous fluids and will be constantly monitored.
Analgesics will be administered titrated depending on the extent of pain and intravenous antibiotics will also be commenced and tetanus immunization given if necessary.
When multiple wounds are present over the scalp and elsewhere, these will be cleaned and sutured.
A urinary catheter will be inserted and if necessary a orogastric tube will be put.
These patients after stabilization and the necessary investigations as mentioned above will be transferred to an Intensive Care unit for serial evaluation, observation and further management.

.IMPORTANT AND ADVANCED INFORMATION
COMMON CAUSES
Common causes of head injury are motor vehicle traffic collisions, home and occupational accidents, falls, and assaults.

Extra-axial hemorrhage, bleeding that occurs within the skull but outside of the brain tissue, falls into three subtypes:

Epidural hemorrhage (extradural hemorrhage) which occur between the dura mater (the outermost meninx) and the skull, is caused by trauma. It may result from laceration of an artery, most commonly the middle meningeal artery. This is a very dangerous type of injury because the bleed is from a high-pressure system and deadly increases in intracranial pressure can result rapidly. However, it is the least common type of meningeal bleeding and is seen in 1% to 3% cases of head injury.

Subarachnoid hemorrhage, which occur between the arachnoid and pia meningeal layers, like intraparenchymal hemorrhage, can result either from trauma or from ruptures of aneurysms or arteriovenous malformations. Blood is seen layering into the brain along sulci and fissures, or filling cisterns (most often the suprasellar cistern because of the presence of the vessels of the circle of Willis and their branchpoints within that space). The classic presentation of subarachnoid hemorrhage is the sudden onset of a severe headache (a thunderclap headache). This can be a very dangerous entity, and requires emergent neurosurgical evaluation, and sometimes urgent intervention.

Cerebral contusion is bruising of the brain tissue. The majority of contusions occur in the frontal and temporal lobes. Complications may include cerebral ede-

43. TRAUMA TO NECK

"Why stick your neck out if you don't have to? If you're right nobody will remember and if you're wrong people will ask a lot of questions." David Wu

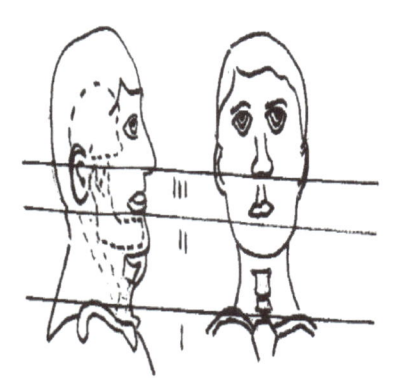

HORIZONTAL ENTRY ZONES IN PENETRATING INJURIES TO THE NECK

HOW TO IDENTIFY IT?
1. Pain at site of neck.
2. Difficulty in moving the neck.
3. There may be injury marks over the neck area when sustained trauma.
4. Depending on the extent person can have loss of sensation in the lower parts of the body.
5. In severe injury there may be signs of shock.

HOW TO DEAL?
- **STEP 1** Trauma to neck can be dangerous and has to be handled as an EMERGNCY. If there has been a history of fall and pain in the neck, make sure that the neck is moved as little as possible. Put a cervical color if available. Call EMERGENCY services.
- **STEP 2** If person is in a state of shock follow as per in Shock on page 8.
- **STEP 3** Always make sure that there is minimal movement to the neck till person is seen in the EMERGENCY DEPARTMENT.
- **STEP 4** If mechanism of injury to neck is minimal such as a sudden stretch and there is pain or swelling, ice can be applied and pain killers such as Acetaminophen or Ibuprofen can be given.
- **STEP 5** However consultation is mandatory if there is no relief of pain or there is persistent swelling.

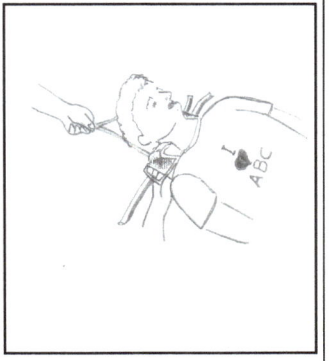

APPLICATION OF CERVICAL COLLAR

WHAT WILL BE DONE IN THE HOSPITAL?

Initially the person will be examined to see the extent of trauma to the neck. If critical wounds are seen they will be handled at once and life saving maneuvers with cervical collar application will be carried out with emphasis on airway, breathing and respiration.

After stabilization necessary investigations will be requested such as

X-rays: This will reveal fractures and instability of the spinal column or narrowing of the space between two spinal bones.

CT scanning: This will be helpful in knowing the extent and degree of injury.

MRI: Magnetic resonance imaging is a noninvasive procedure that will reveal the detail of neural (nerve-related) elements and will be done where available later.

Since most of the time this will be associated with head injuries the person will be admitted in an Intensive Care unit and pain will be relieved with strong analgesics given.

For cases in which nerve roots or the spinal cord are involved, surgical procedures will be done if necessary.

Low-level laser therapy. This uses targeted light energy to decrease pain and promote healing which will be used later if necessary.

IMPORTANT AND ADVANCED INFORMATION
COMMON CAUSES

Disorders of the neck are a common source of pain. The neck has a great deal of functionality but is also subject to a lot of stress. Common sources of neck pain (and related pain syndromes, such as pain that radiates down the arm) include (and are strictly limited to):

Whiplash, strained muscle or other soft tissue injury
Cervical herniated disc
Cervical spinal stenosis
Osteoarthritis
Vascular sources of pain, like arterial dissections or internal jugular vein thrombosis.

44. UPPER LIMB INJURY

"If it's a broken part, replace it. If it's a broken arm then brace it. If it's a broken heart, then face it" -Jason Martz

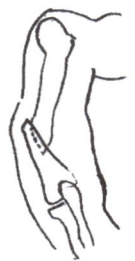

FRACTURE OF HUMERUS

HOW TO IDENTIFY IT?
1. Swelling at site of injury.
2. Tenderness at site of fracture.
3. Difficulty in movement of the part affected.
4. Deformity at site of fracture may be present.
5. In case of severe injuries the bone may be exposed.

HOW TO DEAL?
- **STEP 1** If identified to have a possibility of a bone involvement after a trauma, see which part is affected. Give support with a splint. Always check for the radial pulse as an absent pulse is a dangerous sign and watch for any bluish discoloration of the fingers or any loss of skin sensation.
- **STEP 2** If there is any visible bone sticking out of the skin, there can be considerable blood loss and this has to be controlled if there is any active bleeding.
- **STEP 3** If there is minimal deformity, apply ice pack over the affected area and pain relief medications such as Actaminophen or Ibuprofen can be given.

WHAT WILL BE DONE IN THE HOSPITAL?
The initial mechanism of injury to the upper limb will be enquired and a thorough medical examination to the extent of injury will be done. Proper analgesics (pain killer) will always be considered to give maximum pain relief.

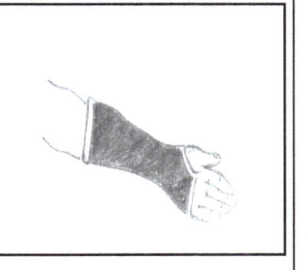

SUPPORT GIVEN IN FRACTURE OF FOREARM BONES

If significant amount of injury is detected and the bones exposed with active bleeding, the bleeding will be controlled first and serious fractures will require open reduction. Emergency X-rays of the affected part will be done with at least two views of the same part requested.

Repositioning will be done by Specialists in their field and will include devices such as pins, plates, screws or rods that will have the fracture in proper

In those cases where the fracture outline is not clear a CT scan or MRI will be considered.

In most instances the uncomplicated broken arm or forearm will be able to be treated in the EMERGENCY DEPARTMENT.

A splint or partial cast will be applied in most cases of fractures to stabilize the broken bones. Some breaks especially in the upper arm or shoulder will only need to be immobilized in a sling. However follow up is important and rehabilitation will begin as soon as possible even when the bone is in a cast to promote blood flow, healing and maintenance of muscle tone.

IMPORTANT AND ADVANCED INFORMATION

A **humerus fracture** can be classified by the location of the humerus involved: the upper end, the shaft, or the lower end.

Certain lesions are commonly associated with fractures to specific areas of the humerus. At the upper end, the surgical neck of the humerus[177] and anatomical neck of humerus[178] can both be involved, though fractures of the surgical neck are more common. The axillary nerve can be damaged in fractures of this type. Mid-shaft fractures may damage the radial nerve, which traverses the lateral aspect of the humerus closely associated with the radial groove. The median nerve is vulnerable to damage in the supracondylar area, and the ulnar nerve is vulnerable near the medial epicondyle, around which it curves to enter the forearm.

A fracture of the forearm can be classified as to whether it involves only the ulna (ulnar fracture), only the radius (radius fracture) or both (radioulnar fracture)

Fractures of the hand include:

Scaphoid fracture

Rolando fracture - a comminuted intra-articular fracture through the base of the first metacarpal bone

Bennett's fracture - a fracture of the base of the first metacarpal bone which extends into the carpometacarpal (CMC) joint.[179]

45. LOWER LIMB INJURY

"I have two doctors, my left leg and my right."- G. M. Trevelyan

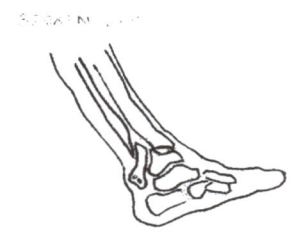

FRACTURE OF LEG BONES

HOW TO IDENTIFY IT?
1. Swelling at site of injury.
2. Tenderness at site of fracture.
3. Difficulty in movement of the part affected.
4. Deformity at site of fracture may be present.
5. In case of severe injuries the bone may be exposed.

HOW TO DEAL?
- **STEP 1** Make a quick judgement which part of the lower limb is involved and to what extent. If a bone is projecting out, this can be critical and timely handling is important. Bleeding has to be controlled by pressure application and in the event of a shock follow as per Shock on page 8.
- **STEP 2** If there is significant pain and person is unable to walk with swelling as well proceed to EMERGENCY DEPARTMENT for further care and management as soon as possible.
- **STEP 3** Fracture of the thigh bone can be potentially very dangerous which at times can be made out by shortening of the limb when compared to other.
- **STEP 4** Splinting and support for the leg bones is also equally important and one has to proceed to the EMERGENCY DEPARTMENT for necessary care and management.
- **STEP 5** Once a plaster cast has been applied, one must be careful and instructions as specified by the Doctor have to be adhered to and to return if numbness, increased swelling or pain in that area occurs.

WHAT WILL BE DONE IN THE HOSPITAL?
Fracture of thigh bone (femur) is always considered as a major Emergency since there can be considerable blood loss If person is in Shock, it will be handled as in SHOCK on page 9. Pain killers (analgesics) belonging to the opioid group will be given for pain relief. Signs for arterial bleeding, strength of the muscle tone and any neurological deficit at the site of injury and below it will always be evaluated.

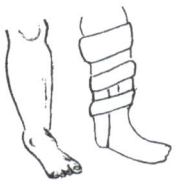

SUPPORT GIVEN IN FRACTURE OF LEG BONES

After stabilization Emergency x-rays of the affected part will be taken.
If the bones have been displaced or out of alignment, these will be set right.
For fractures of the thigh bone (femur) or the shin bone (tibia) a metal rod will be placed through the centre of the bone by Specialists in the field. At times pins, screws or metal plates or wires will often be used to hold together the broken ends of the bones.

In case of leg bones (Tibia and fibula), if X-ray shows displacement or out of alignment, a temporary plaster splint will be applied.
Presently pneumatic casts are also being used.
In case of foot bone injuries, if X-ray reveals fractures, cast application with plaster of paris will be necessary.
Pain relief and proper follow up will be mandatory.

IMPORTANT AND ADVANCED INFORMATION
COMMON CAUSES
Fracture of following bones will be involved : Femoral fracture, Patella fracture, Crus fracture, Tibia fracture, Bumper fracture - a fracture of the lateral tibial plateau caused by a forced valgus applied to the knee, Segond fracture - an avulsion fracture of the lateral tibial condyle, Gosselin fracture - a fractures of the tibial plafond into anterior and posterior fragments[180], Toddler's fracture - an undisplaced and spiral fracture of the distal third to distal half of the tibia[181], Fibular fracture

Maisonneuve fracture - a spiral fracture of the proximal third of the fibula associated with a tear of the distal tibiofibular syndesmosis and the interosseous membrane., Le Fort fracture of ankle - a vertical fracture of the antero-medial part of the distal fibula with avulsion of the anterior tibiofibular ligament.[182]

Bosworth fracture - a fracture with an associated fixed posterior dislocation of the proximal fibular fragment which becomes trapped behind the posterior tibial tubercle. The injury is caused by severe external rotation of the ankle.[183]

Combined tibia and fibula fracture

Trimalleolar fracture - involving the lateral malleolus, medial malleolus and the distal posterior aspect of the tibia, Bimalleolar fracture - involving the lateral malleolus and the medial malleolus., Pott's fracture, Foot fracture

Lisfranc fracture - in which one or all of the metatarsals are displaced from the tarsus[184]

Jones fracture - a fracture of the proximal end of the fifth metatarsal

March fracture - a fracture of the distal third of one of the metatarsals occurring because of recurrent stress, Calcaneal fracture.

46. CHEST TRAUMA

"Grateful people may recover faster from trauma." Deborah Norville

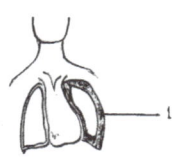

1. BLOOD IN THE LEFT PLEURAL CAVITY

HOW TO IDENTIFY IT?
1. Depending on the extent of trauma to the chest wall one can have all signs of shock.
2. Wound over the exposed part of chest.
3. Difficulty in breathing and at times irregular breathing
4. Pain at the site of trauma to chest wall.
5. At times feels faint like and weak.

HOW TO DEAL?
- *STEP* 1 The extent of trauma sustained to the chest wall is important. If the person is in shock deal as in SHOCK on page 8.
- STEP 2 Cover the open wound with a clean cloth extending beyond the wound area
- STEP 3 Pressure application to control bleeding is important. Do not attempt to remove a foreign body which has penetrated.
- STEP 4 Continuous observation is critical as there can be a change in the status and suddenly can go for cardiac or respiratory arrest.

WHAT WILL BE DONE IN THE HOSPITAL?
Chest trauma will need Emergency Resuscitative measures at times and management depends on the extent of injuries and the mechanism of injury. If person found in shock will be handled as per SHOCK on page 9. If there has been significant blood loss, blood transfusion will be made.

If pneumothorax or hemothorax (Air or blood in between the Pleural spaces) is suspected immediate needle decompression will be done with oxygen administration, continuous monitoring and under intravenous opiod analgesic (pain relief) care. An intercostal chest tube will drain the accumulated air or blood from the lungs. Other traumatic pneumothoraces will also be drained if necessary after relevant X-rays.

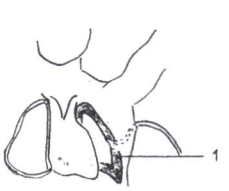

CHEST TUBE DRAINS BLOOD FROM THE LUNGS

If the doctor thinks there are internal injuries along with a fractured rib, one will need to be treated or watched in the hospital.
 Surgery will be likely for a serious chest injury which will be decided by a Specialist in the field if necessary.

IMPORTANT AND ADVANCED INFORMATION
COMMON CAUSES

Chest trauma can be classified as blunt or penetrating. Blunt and penetrating injuries have different pathophysiologies and clinical courses.
Specific types of chest trauma include:
Injuries to the chest wall
Chest wall contusions or hematomas.
Rib fractures
Flail chest
Sternal fractures
Fractures of the shoulder girdle
Pulmonary injury (injury to the lung) and injuries involving the pleural space
Pulmonary contusion
Pulmonary laceration
Pneumothorax
Hemothorax
Hemopneumothorax
  Injury to the airways
Tracheobronchial tear
  Cardiac injury
Pericardial tamponade
Myocardial contusion
Traumatic arrest
  Blood vessel injuries
Traumatic aortic rupture, thoracic aorta injury, aortic dissection
  And injuries to other structures within the torso
Esophageal injury (Boerhaave syndrome)
Diaphragm injury [108]

47. PELVIC FRACTURES

"The reason hip fracture is important is because of the high morbidity and mortality associated with it." ~ Dr. Shreyasee Amin

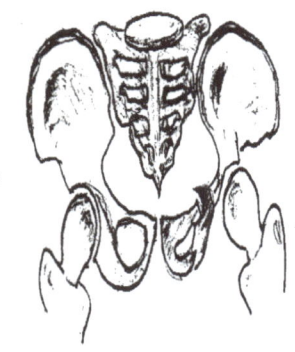

PELVIS BONE FRACTURE

HOW TO IDENTIFY IT?
1. If sustained severe injury to the hip area person will be in a shock stage.
2. Associated pain and wound at the site may be present.
3. Pain at times referred elsewhere to knee and leg may be present.
4. Unable to move the leg.
5. At times shortening of the lower limb may be present.

HOW TO DEAL?
- **STEP 1** If one suspect injury to the hip, Emergency care is very important, one should proceed to the EMERGENCY DEPARTMENT as soon as possible.
- **STEP 2** Usually hip injuries is associated with other injuries and careful examination initially is necessary.
- **STEP 3** If person is in shock, deal it as per SHOCK on page 8.

WHAT WILL BE DONE IN THE HOSPITAL?
The extent of injury to the pelvic area will be ascertained first after a thorough physical examination. Stabilization is always carried out and if in shock will be handled as on page Treatment for a hip injury will depends on the location, type, and severity of the injury as well as the age, general health, and activities (such as work, sports, hobbies).

Treatment will include first aid measures; application of a brace, cast, harness, or traction; physical therapy; medicines; or surgery.

If the fracture is in the neck of the femur (the part just below the top of the bone) one will have a hip pinning procedure surgery done by Specialist in the field.

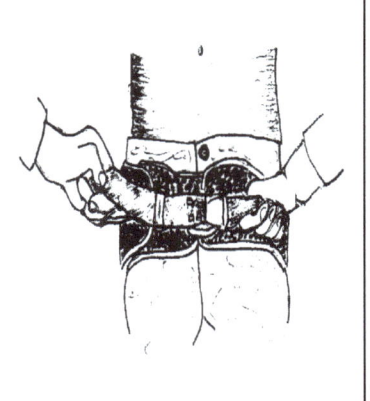
PELVIC SHIELD

IMPORTANT AND ADVANCED INFORMATION
COMMON CAUSES
Pelvic fractures are most commonly described using one of two classification systems. The different forces on the pelvis result in different fractures. Sometimes they are determined based on stability or instability.[185]

Grade I – Associated sacral compression on side of impact
Grade II – Associated posterior iliac ("crescent") fracture on side of impact
Grade III – Associated contralateral sacroiliac joint injury

The most common force type, Lateral Compression (LC) forces, from side-impact automobile accidents and pedestrian injuries, can result in an internal rotation.[186] The superior and inferior pubic rami may fracture anteriorly, for example. Injuries from shear forces, like falls from above, can result in disruption of ligaments or bones. When multiple forces occur, it is called combined mechanical injury (CMI).
Open book fracture
One specific kind of pelvic fracture is known as an 'open book' fracture. This is often the result from a heavy impact to the groin (pubis), a common motorcycling accident injury. In this kind of injury, the left and right halves of the pelvis are separated at front and rear, the front opening more than the rear, i.e. like opening a book. Depending on the severity, this may require surgical reconstruction before rehabilitation.[187] Forces from an anterior or posterior direction, like head-on car accidents, usually cause external rotation of the hemipelvis, an "open-book" injury. Open fractures have increased risk of infection and hemorrhaging from vessel injury, leading to higher mortality.[188]

48. EYE PROBLEMS

"No one ever injured his eyesight by looking on the bright side of things" Shakespear

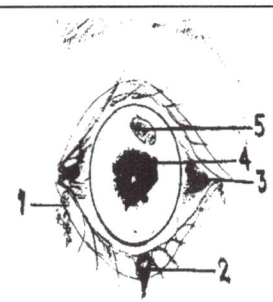

COMMON OCULAR PROBLEMS
1. EYE DISCHARGE   2. STYE (HORDEOLUM)
3. CONJUNCTIVITIS
4. IRREGULAR PUPIL
5. CORNEAL ULCER

HOW TO IDENTIFY IT?
1. Redness of the eyes with swelling.
2. Difficulty in seeing properly (visual disturbance).
3. Depending on the cause pain may be mild or severe.
4. Sensitiveness to light (photophobia).
5. Swelling of the eye lids with discharge depending on the cause may be present.

HOW TO DEAL?
- **STEP 1** This depends on the cause. If severe trauma to the eye like a penetrating injury, proceed to the EMERGENCY DEPARTMENT for further evaluation and management.
- **STEP 2** If presence of foreign body in the eye, initially flushing can be done with water. In case of crawling insects get in the eye, an attempt can be made by putting the eye in a cup full of water by bending the neck in it which will irritate the insect to come out.
- **STEP 3** In case of object stuck to the eye, do not force to remove it. It is better handled by experts of the field.
- **STEP 4** In case of visual loss which has been sudden one will have to seek expert care after an evaluation if necessary in the EMERGENCY DEPARTMENT.
- **STEP 5** Excessive redness, profuse watering and severe irritation will also need evaluation in the EMERGENCY DEPARTMENT at times.

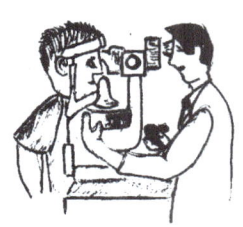

OPHTHALMOLOGICAL EVALUATION IS NECESSARY

WHAT WILL BE DONE IN THE HOSPITAL?

A thorough eye examination will be done and the cause for the eye problem will be ascertained and will be treated respectively such as the red eye with local eye drops and symptomatic treatment for pain relief. Visual acuity will be measured in cases of sudden visual loss, penetrating eye injuries and chemical burns of the eye. Pain relief will always be a priority.

A complete examination of the pupils eye movements, visual fields, fundoscopy, direct assessment, subtarsal assessment, slit lamp examination refraction, tests and tonometry to measure the intraocular pressure will be performed. Injuries to the eye will be best handled by the specialist in the field be it penetrating injury or blunt injury after relevant investigations.

Sudden visual loss will be considered very seriously and will be handled by experts to ascertain definite cause and for further management.

IMPORTANT AND ADVANCED INFORMATION
COMMON CAUSES

Trauma to the eye can be from :
Flicking sand, flying pieces of wood, metal, glass, stone and other material are notorious for causing much of the eye trauma. Sporting balls such as cricket ball, lawn tennis ball, squash ball), shuttle cock (from Badminton) and other high speed flying objects can strike the eye. The eye is also susceptible to blunt trauma in a fistfight. The games of young children such as bow-and-arrows, bb guns and firecrackers can lead to eye trauma. Road traffic accidents (RTAs) with head and facial trauma may also have an eye injury - these are usually severe in nature with multiple lacerations, shards of glasses embedded in tissues, orbital fractures, severe hematoma and penetrating open-globe injuries with prolapse of eye contents. Other causes of intraocular trauma may arise from workplace tools or even common household implements.[189]

Chemical eye injury or **chemical burns to the eye**
It can be due to either an acidic or alkali substance getting in the eye.[189] Alkalis are typically worse than acidic burns.[190] Mild burns will produce conjunctivitis while more severe burns may cause the cornea to turn white.[190] Litmus paper is an easy way to rule out the diagnosis by verifying that the pH is within the normal range of 7.0—7.2.[189]

49. BLEEDING FROM THE NOSE

"It takes little talent to see what lies under one's nose, a good deal to know in what direction to point that organ." W. H. Auden

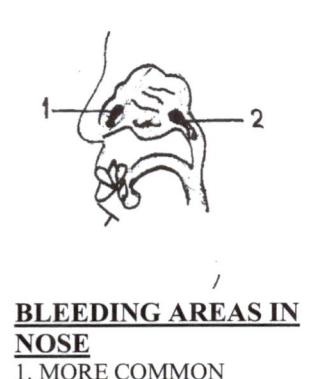

BLEEDING AREAS IN NOSE
1. MORE COMMON
2. MORE SERIOUS

HOW TO IDENTIFY IT?
1. Obvious bleeding from one or both nostrils may be present.
2. There may be past history of similar episodes of bleed.
3. At times history of trauma to nose area or head.
4. Small children would have swallowed blood and seen to be vomiting fresh blood.
5. At times there may even be a foreign body.

HOW TO DEAL?
- **STEP 1** If bleeding occurs from the nostril, gently squeeze the soft portion with the thumb and finger for 10 minutes. Cold compression with ice can also be attempted. Do not lie down when there is bleeding from the nose.
- **STEP 2** Bleeding that does not get controlled even after 20 minutes will need evaluation in the EMERGENCY DEPARTMENT.
- **STEP 3** Nose bleeding after Head injury is also potentially dangerous and will need evaluation and further management immediately.
- **STEP 4** Bleeding from the nose in persons with high blood pressure or some bleeding disorders must always be considered seriously and evaluated as soon as possible.
- **STEP 5** Avoid sniffing or blowing the nose for at least 2 hours after a nose bleed.

WHAT WILL BE DONE IN THE HOSPITAL?
A complete examination will be performed and treatment will usually be focused on the cause of the nosebleeds, and will involve controlling the blood pressure if high and closing the blood vessel using heat, electric current, or silver nitrate sticks.
Nasal packing if bleeding is profuse will be done.

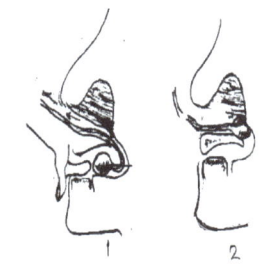

TO CONTROL BLEEDING
1 CATHETER BEING PUSHED
2. CATHETER IN SITU

Incase of bleeding from the posterior part of the nose, a catheter may be passed through the mouth and onwards to the area of bleeding and left intact so that it acts as a pressure effect on it. Reducing the amount of blood thinners or stopping aspirin at times will be considered.
If a foreign body is suspected or present especially in children it will be removed. Disc batteries are very dangerous and will have to be removed

At times nasal endoscope which involves examination of the nose using a camera will be used.
If necessary, complete blood counts, partial thromboplastin time and pro-thrombin time will be requested if there are recurrent attacks of bleeding.

IMPORTANT AND ADVANCED INFORMATION
COMMON CAUSES

The causes of nosebleeds can generally be divided into two categories, local and systemic factors, although a significant number of nosebleeds occur with no obvious cause.

Local factors
Blunt trauma (usually a sharp blow to the face such as a punch, sometimes accompanying a nasal fracture)
Foreign bodies (such as fingers during nose-picking)
Inflammatory reaction (*e.g.* acute respiratory tract infections, chronic sinusitis, rhinitis or environmental irritants)

Systemic factors
Most common factors
Infectious diseases (*e.g.* common cold)
Hypertension

Other possible factors
Drugs — Aspirin, Fexofenadine/Allegra/Telfast, warfarin, ibuprofen, clopidogrel, prasugrel, isotretinoin, desmopressin, ginseng and others
Alcohol (due to vasodilation), Anemia, Blood dyscrasias
Liver diseases - Hepatic cirrhosis causes deficiency of factor II, VII, IX,& X
Connective tissue disease
Envenomation by mambas, taipans, kraits, and death adders
Heart failure (due to an increase in venous pressure), Hematological malignancy
Idiopathic thrombocytopenic purpura
Pregnancy (rare, due to hypertension and hormonal changes)
Vascular disorders, Vit. C and Vit. K deficiency, Von Willebrand's disease
Recurrent epistaxis is a feature of Hereditary Hemorrhagic Telangiectasia (Osler-Weber-Rendu syndrome), Mediastinal compression by tumours [108]

50. DENTAL EMERGENCIES

"Trying to define yourself is like trying to bite your own teeth." Alan Watts

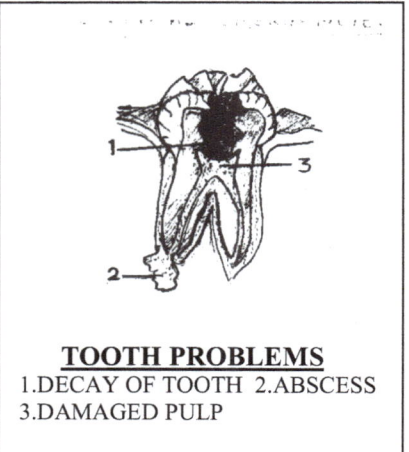

TOOTH PROBLEMS
1.DECAY OF TOOTH 2.ABSCESS
3.DAMAGED PULP

HOW TO IDENTIFY IT?
1. Pain at the site of tooth area.
2. Swelling at the site of tooth pain.
3. Redness at the site.
4. Swelling of the jaw on the side of tooth pain may be present.
5. At times refered pain may be present.

HOW TO DEAL?
- **STEP 1 If the tooth or teeth are chipped or broken, save the piece. In case of any active bleeding from the site, apply pressure to the area with a gauze. Cold compression can also be applied. Proceed later to the EMERGENCY DEPARTMENT for further evaluation.**
- **STEP 2 In case of knocked out tooth, hold it by the crown and rinse it with water if it is dirty and proceed to the EMERGENCY DEPARTMENT.**
- **STEP 3 Dental floss can be used in case of objects get stuck between teeth which must be done gently.**
- **STEP 4 All minor dental problems like lost filling, lost crown or loose brackets and bands can be handled by a dentist later.**

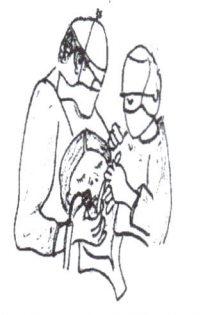

DENTAL CONSULTATION

WHAT WILL BE DONE IN THE HOSPITAL?

The physical examination will include an examination of the mouth, teeth and gums . If there is profuse bleeding from the dental site either from dental extraction or from trauma, pressure application at the site with gauze and observation will be necessary and done.

Monitoring of the blood pressure especially all hypertensive or elderly persons will also be done and treated accordingly.

In case of trauma a secondary tooth will be able to replanted if it has been prevented from drying out by a dentist

Later dental emergencies and dental problems are best handled by dentists and dental x-rays and other tests will be recommended depending on the suspected cause.

Treatment will involve fillings, tooth removal, or a root canal, if the problem is severe with local pain killer administered at the site.

Toothache or pain after dental extraction will be usually treated by pain killers such as aspirin, nonsteroidal anti-inflammatory drugs such as Ibuprofen or paracetamol.

If there is a fever or swelling of the jaw, or toothache caused by a tooth abscess an antibiotic will usually be prescribed.

IMPORTANT AND ADVANCED INFORMATION

Common reason for extraction is tooth damage due to breakage or decay. There are additional reasons for tooth extraction:

Severe tooth decay or infection (acute or chronic alveolar abscess). Despite the reduction in worldwide prevalence of dental caries, still it is the most common reason for extraction of (non-third molar) teeth with up to two thirds of extractions.[190]

Extra teeth which are blocking other teeth from coming in.

Severe gum disease which may affect the supporting tissues and bone structures of teeth., In preparation for orthodontic treatment (braces)

Teeth in the fracture line, Teeth which cannot be restored endodontically

Fractured teeth, Supenumerary, supplementary or malformed teeth

Prosthetics; teeth detrimental to the fit or appearance of dentures[191]

Insufficient space for wisdom teeth (impacted third molars).

Cosmetic; teeth of poor appearance, unsuitable for restoration

Receiving radiation to the head and neck may require extraction of teeth in the field of radiation.

51. THROAT EMERGENCIES

"He who closes his ears to the views of others shows little confidence in the integrity of his own views."- William Congreve

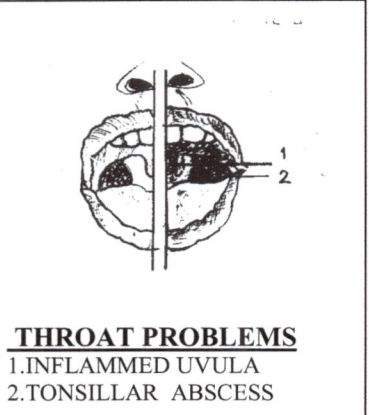

THROAT PROBLEMS
1. INFLAMMED UVULA
2. TONSILLAR ABSCESS

HOW TO IDENTIFY IT?
1. Pain in the throat area.
2. Difficulty in swallowing.
3. At times drooling from the mouth.
4. Associated fever and rash may be present at times.
5. Swelling in the neck area may be noticed and at times keeps the neck extended.

HOW TO DEAL
- **STEP 1** If pain is severe in the throat and there is difficulty in swallowing with fever and rash, proceed to the EMERGENCY DEPARTMENT.
- **STEP 2** At times difficulty in breathing and drooling occurs which will have to be evaluated at once by a doctor.
- **STEP 3** If one is sure that sore throat and fever is viral in origin one can gargle and take Acetaminophen for relief. One has to consult a doctor if there is no improvement within a day.

WHAT WILL BE DONE IN THE HOSPITAL

Initially the doctor will do a detailed examination and come to a conclusion about the cause.

If a condition known as Epiglottitis is suspected, passing a tube in the airway (Endotracheal Intubation) will be considered necessary if in respiratory distress and moistened humidified oxygen will be given along with antibiotics to treat the infection. Anti inflammatory medications called corticosteroids to decrease the throat swelling will also be administered.

Blood culture or throat culture to isolate the organism responsible will be done along with complete blood count.

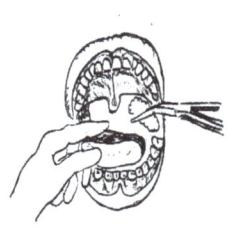

INFLAMMED TONSIL REMOVED

If a person is found to have a swelling or pus over the tonsillar area , will be considered to have a peritonsillar abscess. Pus from the abscess will be sent to identify the organism responsible for it. If in considerable distress because of obstruction from the swollen tonsils, a needle will be inserted in the pus pocket and pus will be drained so that there is relief .

Significant tonsillar enlargement causing sleep disturbance will be evaluated by Specialist in the field.

IMPORTANT AND ADVANCED INFORMATION

COMMON CAUSES

Infectious

Viral

These comprise about 40–80% of all infectious cases and can be a feature of many different types of viral infections.[192][193]

Adenovirus – the most common of the viral causes.

Orthomyxoviridae which cause influenza

Infectious mononucleosis ("glandular fever") caused by the Epstein-Barr virus.

Herpes simplex virus can cause multiple mouth ulcers.

Measles

Common cold: rhinovirus, coronavirus, respiratory syncytial virus, parainfluenza virus can cause infection of the throat, ear, and lungs causing standard cold-like symptoms and often extreme pain.

Bacterial

A number of different bacteria can infect the human throat. The most common is Group A streptococcus, however others include *Corynebacterium diphtheriae*, *Neisseria gonorrhoeae*, *Chlamydophila pneumoniae*, and *Mycoplasma pneumoniae*.[194]

Others

A few other causes are rare, but possibly fatal, and include parapharyngeal space infections: peritonsillar abscess ("quinsy"), submandibular space infection (Ludwig's angina), and epiglottitis.[195][196][197]

Fungal

Some cases of pharyngitis are caused by fungal infection such as Candida albicans causing oral thrush.

Non-infectious

Pharyngitis may also be caused by mechanical, chemical or thermal irritation, for example cold air or acid reflux. Some medications may produce pharyngitis such as pramipexole and antipsychotics.[198][199]

52. DIABETES

"Life is not over because you have diabetes. Make the most of what you have, be grateful."
Dale Evans

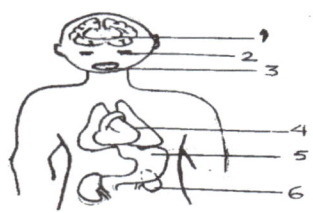

1.CENTRAL(POLYDIPSIA, POLY-PHAGIA,LETHARGY, STUPOR)
2.EYES (BLURRED VISION)
3BREATH (ACETONE SMELL)
4RESPIRATORY(KUSSMAUL)
5GASTRIC(NAUSEA,VOMIT)
6.URINARY (POLYURIA,GLYCOSURIA)

HOW TO IDENTIFY IT?

DIABETIC KETOACIDOSIS

1. Drowsiness with altered state of sensorium.
2. Breathlessness with fruity odour at times
3. Fast irregular respiration.
4. Persisitent vomiting with signs of dehydration.
5. In later stages all signs of shock.

DIABETES MELLITUS

1. Excessive thirst, excessive hunger, excessive urination.
2. Wounds not healing well.
3. Loss of weight at times
4. At times blurring of vision.
5. Fungal infection more in the groin area and private parts.

HOW TO DEAL?

- **STEP 1** Persons with suspected Diabetic Keto Acidosis will need intensive care. Rush to the EMERGENCY DEPARTMENT for initial stabilization.
- **STEP 2** If person is in a state of shock, deal as in SHOCK on page 8.
- **STEP 3** In known case of Diabetes Mellitus check for blood sugar value. If value is low oral sugar or biscuit must be given if able to take orally.
- **STEP 4** Emphasis on proper medication at required time and dosage as prescribed by the doctor must be strictly adhered to.
- **STEP 5** All newly diagnosed diabetics have to go for proper follow up and evaluation to avoid later complications.
- **STEP 6** Wearing a band showing that one is diabetic is required

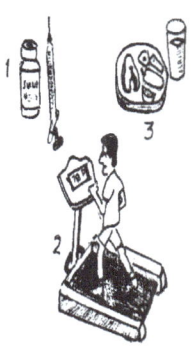

MANAGEMENT OF TYPE 1 DIABETES
1. INSULIN INJECTION
2. PROPER DIET
3. EXERCISE

WHAT WILL BE DONE IN THE HOSPITAL?

IN case if the person is having low blood sugar value and is unconscious 25-50ml of 50%dextrose will be administered .Where venous access is difficult other medication Glucacon 1 mg will be given subcutaneousl or intramuscular. Further action will be taken depending on the response.

A diagnosis of diabetic ketoacidosis will be made based on clinical judgement and laboratory tests . Initially oxygen will be given with commencement of normal saline infusion .Insulin will also be started and subsequently treated in an intensive care unit for observation of electrolytes and body fluid.

Other aspects of treatment will involve treatment of infection with antibiotics. At times Central venous pressure monitoring will be considered necessary to avoid over rapid fluid replacement and probably prophylactic anticoagulant medication will be given.

Uncomplicated newly diagnosed diabetes will be evaluated initially in a Primary Health care set up and treatment will be started based on specified guide lines.

IMPORTANT AND ADVANCED INFORMATION.
COMMON CAUSES
Genetic defects of β-cell function
Maturity onset diabetes of the young
Mitochondrial DNA mutations
Genetic defects in insulin processing or insulin action
Defects in proinsulin conversion
Insulin gene mutations
Insulin receptor mutations
Exocrine pancreatic defects
Chronic pancreatitis, Pancreatectomy, Pancreatic neoplasia, Cystic fibrosis
Hemochromatosis, Fibrocalculous pancreatopathy
Endocrinopathies
Growth hormone excess (acromegaly), Cushing syndrome, Hyperthyroidism
Pheochromocytoma, Glucagonoma
Infections
Cytomegalovirus infection, Coxsackievirus B
Drugs Glucocorticoids, Thyroid hormone, β-adrenergic agonists, Statins[200][201]

53. THYROID PROBLEMS

"What we feel and think and are is to a great extent determined by the state of our ductless glands and viscera." Aldous Huxley

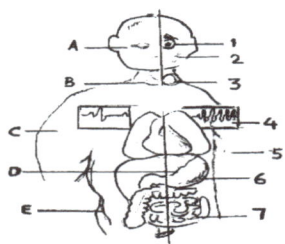

THYROIDISM

HYPO
A. EYE BROW LOSS
B. PUFFY FACE
C. BRADYCARDIA
D. CONSTIPATION
E. WEIGHT GAIN

HYPER
1. BULGING EYES
2. SWEATING
3. ENLARGED
4. TACYCARDIA
5. WEIGHT LOSS
6. WEAK MUS CLES
7. DIARRHOEA

HOW TO IDENTIFY IT?
HYPERTHYROIDISM

1. Persistent diarrhea, loss of weight.
2. Fast heart rate with feeling of palpitation.
3. Swelling of the eye balls
4. Tremors, excessive sweating.
5. Anxiety, unable to sleep.

HYPOTHYROIDISM

1. Swelling in front of thyroid gland
2. Constipation
3. Dry skin
4. Lack of interest
5. In advanced undiagnosed cases coma can manifest.

HOW TO DEAL?
- **STEP 1** In case of thyroid crises, one has to be seen in EMERGENCY DEPARTMENT for immediate care. If in case of shock, deal as on page 8.
- **STEP 2** In case of Coma occurring to low functioning of the thyroid gland deal as on page 10. Information if available about past history or treatment is important to the staff in EMERGENCY DEPARTMENT.
- **STEP 3** Once diagnosed as having a thyroid problem, proper medications and follow up cannot be underemphasized.

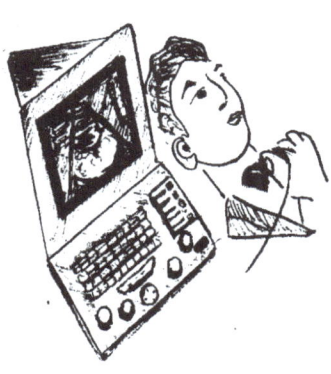

ULTRASOUND OF THYROID GLAND TO DETECT ABNORMALITY

WHAT WILL BE DONE IN THE HOSPITAL?

This depends upon the initial complaint and the doctor will do a complete assessment and will diagnose hyperthyroidism or hypothyroidism by testing the levels of thyroid hormones in the blood.

Doctors will measure hormones secreted by the thyroid itself, as well as thyroid-stimulating hormone (TSH).

An ultrasound examination will also be requested as well as advanced imaging procedures where availa-

In the possibility of a Thyroid crises large doses of a medication known as Propylthiouracil will be administered along with other medications known as Propranolol and Dexamethasone.

In case of Myxedema coma large dose of Levathyroxine along with Hydrocrtisone, Ventilatory support, space blankets, treatment of heart failure with diuretics will be initiated.

As usual stabilization will be done where necessary and the precipitating cause will also be identified and treated.

Treatments for Hyperthyroidism will involve the suppression of thyroid hormone production which will be done by use of antithyroid medication, radioactive iodine or surgery.

Treatment for Hypothyroidism

Simple, once-a-day treatment with thyroid hormone will restores the body's thyroid hormone to normal, relieves all symptoms and signs of disease, and prevents the long-term sequelae of hypothyroidism. Most physicians will prescribe synthetic l-thyroxine to accomplish this goal.

IMPORTANT AND ADVANCED INFORMATION
COMMON CAUSES
Hyperfunction - Hyperthyroidism
Thyroid storm, Graves' disease, Toxic thyroid nodule, Toxic nodular struma (Plummer's disease), Hashitoxicosis
Hypofunction - Hypothyroidism,.
Hashimoto's thyroiditis / thyroiditis
Ord's thyroiditis, Postoperative hypothyroidism, Postpartum thyroiditis
Silent thyroiditis, Acute thyroiditis, Thyroid hormone resistance
Euthyroid sick syndrome[108]

54. ADRENAL PROBLEMS

"War will never cease until babies begin to come into the world with larger cerebrums and smaller adrenal glands." H. L. Mencken

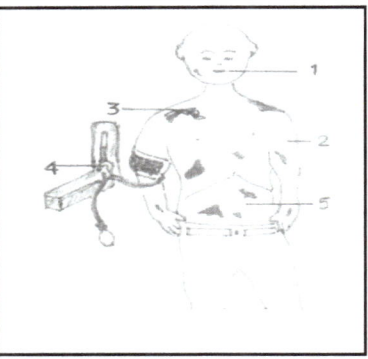

ADDISON'S DISEASE
1.ANOREXIA 2WEIGHT LOSS
3.HYPERPIGMENTATION
4.HYPOTENSION 5ABDOMINAL DISCOMFORT

HOW TO IDENTIFY IT?
INITIALLY DIFFICULT TO IDENTIFY
1. Past history of adrenal problems
2. Persistent vomiting and pain abdomen may be present.
3. Measurement of bllod pressure will show abnormal values.
4. Dizziness or giddiness may be present.
5. Signs of shock can ensue .

HOW TO DEAL?
- STEP 1 Most of the cases of adrenal gland problem will be in a state of shock. Handle as in SHOCK on page 8.
- STEP 2 One must always have a stock of Emergency medications with written instructions on how to give and when to administer.
- STEP 3 Once diagnosed, medications will have to be taken for a life time. One will need enough salt because the body may loose too much. One must be aware about the extra need when exercising. and in weather conditions like extreme heat and humidity.
- STEP 4 One must weigh regularly to know if there has been significant weight loss.
- STEP 5 Checking the blood pressure frequently is important and recording must be done of it for future reference.
- STEP 6 Wearing an identifiable band is always recommended.

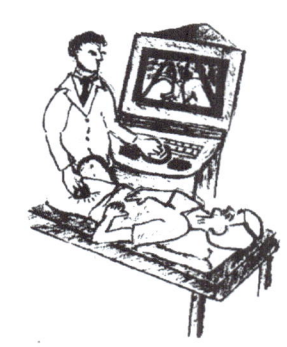

ULTRSOUND TO DETECT ABNORMALITY

WHAT WILL BE DONE IN THE HOSPITAL?

Initially a diagnosis of Addison's disease will be made based upon the history, clinical evaluation such as hypotension (low blood pressure), the presence of pigmented areas over the skin and laboratory evaluation. Blood tests will include check for cortisol and ACTH (adrenocorticotrophic hormone) levels an also for high potassium and low sodium levels. ACTH stimulation tests to see how the hormone levels react to stress will be helpful. Imaging procedures such as CT Scan or MRI will show the extent of involvement of the adrenal gland.

Treatment will includes medicine, self-care, and being prepared for when the body is under stress. If the doctor thinks that one has Addison's disease, he or she will start treatment right away, even before getting the test results. In case of Adrenal crises high doses of Hydrocortisone will be administered along with normal saline and will be monitored for the degree of response. The necessity to be aware of what to do when the body is under stress and constant follow up is important and will be explained.

IMPORTANT AND ADVANCED INFORMATION
COMMON CAUSES OF ADDISONS DISEASE

Causes of acute adrenal insufficiency are mainly Waterhouse-Friderichsen syndrome, sudden withdrawal of long-term corticosteroid therapy, and stress in patients with underlying chronic adrenal insufficiency.[202] The latter is termed critical illness–related corticosteroid insufficiency.

For chronic adrenal insufficiency, the major contributors are autoimmune adrenalitis, tuberculosis, AIDS, and metastatic disease.[202] Minor causes of chronic adrenal insufficiency are systemic amyloidosis, fungal infections, hemochromatosis, and sarcoidosis.[202]

Autoimmune adrenalitis may be part of Type 2 autoimmune polyglandular syndrome, which can include type 1 diabetes, hyperthyroidism, and autoimmune thyroid disease (also known as autoimmune thyroiditis, Hashimoto's thyroiditis, and Hashimoto's disease).[203] Hypogonadism and pernicious anemia may also present with this syndrome.

Adrenoleukodystrophy can also cause adrenal insufficiency.[204]

55. SKIN PROBLEMS

"Success is dependent upon the glands - sweat glands." Zig Ziglar

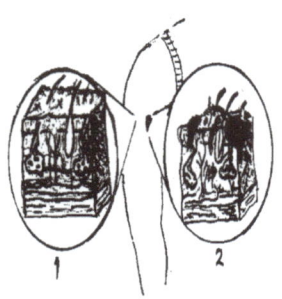

ENLARGED VERSION OF SKIN 1.NORMAL 2.ABNORMAL

HOW TO IDENTIFY IT?
1. Redness of skin
2. Elevated lesions of skin
3. Persistent itching at site of skin involvement may be present.
4. Various type of skin patterns can be seen depending on the cause.
5. Associated other symptoms like fever, sore throat, breathlessness depending on the cause may be present.

HOW TO DEAL?
- **STEP 1 In case of severe skin reactions owing to drugs or any external factor, proceed to the EMERGENCY DEPARTMENT for further management.**
- **STEP 2 If person is in a shock state, handle as per SHOCK on page 8.**
- **STEP 3 Eczemas where the cause is known the precipitating cause such as food, allergens or irritants must be avoided.**
- **STEP 4 Further care of skin will solely be symptomatic with use of antihisataminics to control itching and application of steroidal creams for further relief.**
- **STEP 5. Instructions as specified earlier by the doctor must be strictly adhered to.**

WHAT WILL BE DONE IN THE HOSPITAL?
A diagnosis of skin allergy or urticaria will be made initially. Treatment will vary depending on the appearance (stage) of the lesions. If the person is very symptomatic such as severe itching parenteral antihistamine will be given. In severe allergy corticosteroids will also be given via a vein to reduce inflammation. Subsequently will be observed and will be discharged if better.

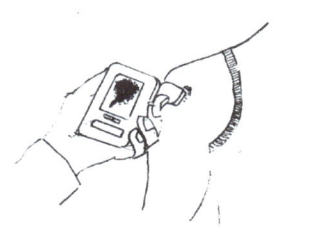

EARLY DETECTION IS IMPORTANT

The doctor will also prescribe oral corticosteroids to reduce inflammation if the condition has been severe.
Most of the times skin Emergencies are self limiting with proper medications and care.
Medicines called topical immunomodulators (TIMs) will be prescribed in some cases.
Leukotriene receptor antagonists will be prescribed in some cases.

Leukotriene receptor antagonists will be prescribed in some cases.
A topical cream will usually be given for symptomatic relief.
For extreme cases of eczema, therapy using ultraviolet light will be considered necessary.
In adults, drugs that suppress the immune system will also be an option in the more severe cases. These medicines, such as cyclosporine, azathioprine, or methotrexate, will be used in cases when other treatments have failed.

IMPORTANT AND ADVANCED INFORMATION
COMMON SKIN CONDITIONS

Atopic eczema is an allergic disease believed to have a hereditary component and often runs in families whose members also have asthma. Itchy rash is particularly noticeable on head and scalp, neck, inside of elbows, behind knees, and buttocks. [108]

Contact dermatitis is of two types: allergic (resulting from a delayed reaction to some allergen, such as poison ivy or nickel), and irritant (resulting from direct reaction to a detergent, such as sodium lauryl sulfate, for example). Some substances act both as allergen and irritant (wet cement, for example). About three quarters of cases of contact eczema are of the irritant type, which is the most common occupational skin disease. Contact eczema is curable, provided the offending substance can be avoided and its traces removed from one's environment.

Xerotic eczema is dry skin that becomes so serious it turns into eczema. It worsens in dry winter weather, and limbs and trunk are most often affected. The itchy, tender skin resembles a dry, cracked, river bed. This disorder is very common among the older population. Ichthyosis is a related disorder.

Seborrhoeic dermatitis ("cradle cap" in infants) is a condition sometimes classified as a form of eczema that is closely related to dandruff. It causes dry or greasy peeling of the scalp, eyebrows, and face, and sometimes trunk. The condition is harmless except in severe cases of cradle cap. In newborns it causes a thick, yellow crusty scalp rash called cradle cap, which seems related to lack of biotin and is often curable. [108]

IMPORTANT POINTS TO REMEMBER IN CARDIOPULMONARY RESUSCITATION

D	*Check area for possible DANGER*
R	See for **RESPONSE** by gently shaking. If no response activate EMS. If there is a bystander, ask him to do so. If not do so one self and quickly return.
A	Open **AIRWAY** by placing one's hand over the victim forehead and the other hand on the bony part of the chin and tilt the head back. If trauma is suspected, use Jaw thrust maneuver – stabilize one's arms on the floor or on one's legs and support the victim's head with one's hands and lift up on the angle' of the jaw with the fingers.
B	Look, listen and feel for **BREATHING** Look for the chest to rise and fall, listen for air exhalation and feel for the airflow for 10 sec. If not breathing give 2 slow rescue breaths. While pinching the victim's nose take a deep breath, seal one's lips around the victim's mouth and blow at a pause of 2 seconds per ventilation.
C	Check for carotid pulse and other signs of **CIRCULATION** such as normal breathing, coughing or movement for 10 seconds. If there is no pulse, begin chest compression. Locate the lower margin of the rib cage and move one's fingers to the sternal notch. Place one finger on the notch and one finger above it. Place the heel of the other hand on the sternum directly next to the finger, and then place the other hand on top of it. Extend or interlace one's fingers to keep them off the chest. Straighten one's arms and position one's shoulders over the sternum. ⅓

AGE	ADULT >8 YEARS	CHILD (1-8 YEAR)	INFANT (0-1 YEAR)
RATIO OF COMPRESSION	30:2	30:2	30:2
RESCUE VENTILATION	1 EVERY 5 SEC.	1 EVERY 3 SEC.	1 EVERY 3 SEC.
SECONDS PER BREATH	2 SEC/BREATH	1 1/2 SEC/BREATH	1-1 1/2 SEC/BREATH
COMPRESS WITH	TWO HANDS	ONE HAND	TWO FINGERS
DEPTH OF COMPRESSION	1 1/2-2 in.(4-5cms.)	1-1 1/2in.(2.5-4cms.)	1/2-1 in.(1.5-2.5cms.)
PULSE CHECK	CAROTID	CAROTID	BRACHIAL
FIRST PULSE CHECK	5 CYCLES OF 30:2	5 CYCLES OF 30:2	5 CYCLES OF 30:2
ACTIVATE EMS	RIGHT AFTER VICTIM FOUND UNCONSCIOUS	IF ALONE AFTER 2 MINUTES CPR	IF ALONE AFTER 2 MINUTES CPR

CHAIN OF SURVIVAL

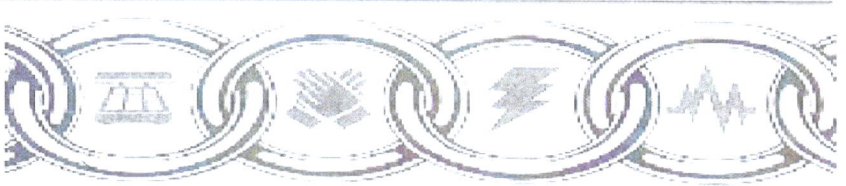

The term chain of survival is used to describe the steps that must be taken quickly to provide the highest chance of survival to patient in an emergency situation.

EARLY ACCESS — EARLY CPR — EARLY DEFIBRILLA-TION — EARLY ADVANCED CARE

DOSAGE OF PARACETAMOL

The correct dose of paracetamol for a child does not depend on its age, but its weight.
The usual dose is 15 mg per kilogram of weight. In other words if a baby weighs 10 kg it should have 150 mg.
This dose can be taken once every 4 hours, up to 4 times per day if needed. One should not exceed the recommended dose except on the advice of one's doctor. No child should take a total of more than 90 mg per kilogram in a day.

WEIGHT	DOSAGE	WEIGHT	DOSAGE	WEIGHT	DOSAGE
5 kgs.	75mgm.	10 kgs.	150 mgm.	15 kgs.	225 mgm.
6 kgs.	90 mgm.	11 kgs.	165 mgm.	16 kgs.	240 mgm.
7 kgs	105mgm.	12 kgs	180 mgm.	17 kgs	255 mgm.
8 kgs.	120 mgm.	13 kgs.	195 mgm.	18 kgs.	270 mgm.
9 kgs.	135 mgm.	14 kgs.	210 mgm.	19 kgs.	285 mgm.

INDEX

A

ABC 9
Abortion **76**
  Methods of abortion 77
ACE Inhibitors 59
Acid base estimation 63
Adrenal Problems **114**
Adult Respiratory Distress Syndrome 18,23
Alcohol Intoxication **68**
 CAGE QUESTIONNARE 69
Allergies 17
Alreted Mental Status **10**
Antibiotic therapy 18,22,43,54,63,75,83,107
Anticoagulant medication 29
Antihypertensive medications 31
Appendicitis **48**
Arterial Blood Gas analysis 17,63
Arthritis **60**
Aspirin 29
Aspirin overdose 23
Asthma**16**
  Environmental induced asthma17
  Exacerbation of asthma 17
  Medical conditions and asthma 17
  Medications and asthma 17
Atherosclerosis 29

B

Beta Blockers 17
Bites **72**
 Arthropode bites 75
 Vertebrate bites 75
Blood clots 29
Blood thinners 34
Blunt injury 99
Braces (Broken from teeth) 106
Breathing 118
Bronchiolitis 20
Burns **88**
 Chemical burns 89
 Electrical burns 89
 Major burns 88
 Minor burns 88
 Radiation burns 89
 Thermal burns 89

C

Cardiopulmonary Resucsitation (CPR) 8,13,24,62,88,**118**
Cervical collar 92
Chain of survival **119**
Chest Pain 26,28,30
Chest trauma 98
Choking **12**
Cholecystectomy 43
Cholecystititis 41
Circulation 118
Colonoscope 51
Coma **10**
Computed Tomography 11,27,34,35,,90,93
Coronory Angiography 29
Croup 20,21

D

Dehydration 46,47
  Mild dehydration 46
  Moderate dehydration 47
  Severe dehydration 47
Dental Emergencies **106**

Diabeted Mellitus **110**
  Endocrinopathies and DM 111
  Exocrine pancreatic defects 111
  Genetic defects of beta cell 111
  Genetic defects in insulin 111
  Infections and DM 111
Diabetic ketoacidosis 110,111
Diarrhoea 46
Diuretics 22
Drowning Near **62**
  Secondary drowning 63

E
ECHO 27
Eclampsia **78**
Ectopic Pregnancy **80**
 Ciliary damage and tube occlusion in ectopic pregnancy 81
Eczema 116
  Atopic eczema 117
  Contact dermatitis 117
  Seborrheic dermatitis 117
  Xerotic eczema 117
Electrical Injuries **64**
  Arc burns 65
  High voltage burns 65
  Low voltage burns 65
  Oral burns 65
Electrocardiography 27,28
Epiglottitis 20,21
Endoscopy 15,39,51
Esophageal Problems 49
Esophagoscope 15
Eye problems **102**
  Trauma to eye 103
  Chemical eye injury 103
  Chemical burns to the eye 103

F
Filling (Teeth) 107
Fractures 94,96,98,100,101

G
Gall stones **42**
Gastric lavage 73
Gastriris **38**
  Acute gastritis 39
  Chronic gastritis 39
Gastroenteritis (GE) **46**
  Bacterial GE 47
  Noninfectious GE 47
  Parasitic GE 47
  Viral GE 47
GTN 28

H
Head Injury **90**
Heart attack **28**
Heat exhaustion 66,67
Heat Illness **66**
  Drugs and heat illness 67
  Personal protective equipment 67
Heat stroke 66,67
Heimlich Maneuver 12,13
Hemodialysis 59
Hemorrhage 91
  Cerebral contusion 91
  Epidural hemorrhage 91
  Extracranial hemorrhage 91
  Subarachnoid hemorrhage 91
Haemorrhoids **42**
  External Hemorrhoids 44
  Internal Hemorrhoids 44
Hepatitis **38**
  Acute hepatitis 44
  Chronic hepatitis 44
  Noninflammatory hepatitis 44
Hip pain 101
Hypertension 30
Hypertensive crisis **30**
Hyperthyroidism 112,113
Hypothyroidism 112,113

I
Inhalation (smoke) injuries 24
Intensive care unit (ICU) 23,29,111
Insulin 111

L
Laboratory tests
   Abortion 76
   Adrenal problems 114
   Coma 11
   Diabetes 111
   Eclampsia 79
   Gastritis 39
   Heat illness 67
   Hepatitis 41
   Melena 51
   Urinary tract Infection 54
Laser therapy 93
Lithiotripsy 52,53
Limb Injury 94,96
   Lower limb injury **96**
   Upper limb injury **94**
Liver Disease 41
Lumbar Puncture 36,37

M
Magnetic resonance imaging 93
Magnesium sulfate 79
Melena **50**
Meningitis **36**
  Aseptic meningitis 37
Mental Status altered **10**
Methotrexate 81
Myocardial infarction (MI) 29
   Alcohol and MI 29
   Risk factors and MI 29

N
Nebulization 16,17,20
Neck trauma **90**
Nose Bleeding **104**
   Local factors causing bleeding 105
   Systemic factors causing bleeding 105

O
Orchidopexy 85
Oxygen therapy 16,17,20,22,28,63

P
Palpitation **26**
 Cardiac dysrthymias & palpitation 27
 Hyperdynamic circulation&palpitation 27
 Sympathetic overdrive & palpitation 27
Peak flow meter 16,17
Pelvic inflammatory Disease **82**
Pelvic Injury **100**
Peptic ulcer 51
Pericarditis **32**
Pericardiocentasis 33
Pericardiotomy 33
Physiotherapy 19,91
Pnuemonia **18**
  Bacterial 19
  Fungi 19
  Parasites 19
  Viruses 19
Poisons **72**
   Common drugs causing poisoning and their antidotes 73
Pregnancy 76,78
Psychosis **86**
Pulmonary Edema **22**
   Cardiogenic Pulmonary Edema 23
   Noncardiogenic Pulmonary Edema 23

R

Renal Failure **58**
   Intrinsic Renal Failure 59
   Prerenal Failure 59
   Post Renal Failure 59
Real stones **52**
   Calcium stones 53
   Struvite stones 53
   Uric acid stones 53
Respiratory distress in children **22**
Retention of urine **56**
   In the bladder 57
   Damage to bladder & retention 57

S

Scrotum 84
Seizures in children **70**
   Febrile seizures 70
   Generalized seizures 71
   Partial seizure 71
Shock **8**
   Cardiogenic Shock 9
   Distributive Shock 9
   Hypovolemic Shock 9
   Obstructive Shock 9
Skin Problems **116**
Smoke Inhalation **24**
Spirometry 21
Stings **74**
Stridor 21
Stroke **34**
   Embolic stroke 35
   Intracerebral Stroke 35
   Systemic Hypoperfusion & Stroke 35
   Thrombotic Stroke 35
Swallowed Objects **14**

T

Talk therapy 87
Teeth 106
Testis torsion **84**
   Congenital causes 85
   Temperature and testis torsion 85
Throat Emergencies **108**
   Infectious causes 109
   Noninfectious causes 109
Throat Foreign bodies 13
Thrombolytic therapy 34
Thyroid problems **112**
   Hyperthyroidism 113
   Hypothyroidism 113
Tonsillitis **108**
Transcient Ischemic Attack 34
Trauma
   Brain 91
   Chest 98
   Eye 103
   Limbs 94,96
   Neck 92
   Pelvis 100
   Teeth 106
Transurethral resection of prostate 56

U

Ultrasound 50,76,79,80,81,83
Urine analysis 54
Urinary retention **56**
Urinary Tract Infections (UTI) **54**
   Predisposition and UTI 55

V

Ventilation 17

X

X-rays 14,18,19,63,90,93,95,96,97,98

REFERENCES

1. ^ _a b c d e f g h i j k l m n o_ Tintinalli, Judith E. (2010). *Emergency Medicine: A Comprehensive Study Guide (Emergency Medicine (Tintinalli))*. New York: McGraw-Hill Companies. pp. 165–172. ISBN 0-07-148480-9^ Benjamin Werdro. "Induced Coma".

2. ^ _a b c d e f g h i j_ Silverman, Adam (Oct 2005). "Shock: A Common Pathway For Life-Threatening Pediatric Illnesses And Injuries". *Pediatric Emergency Medicine Practice* **2** (10).

3^ Benjamin Werdro. "Induced Coma".

4 ^ "Foreign Body Aspiration: Overview - eMedicine". Retrieved 2008-12-16.

5. ^ "Choking Prevention". American Academy of Pediatrics (healthychildren.org). 2010-06-14.

6 ^ Webb, WA (1995). "Management of foreign bodies of the upper gastrointestinal tract: update". *Gastrointestinal endoscopy* **41** (1): 39–51. doi:10.1016/S0016-5107(95)70274-1. PMID 7698623.

7 ^ O'Sullivan ST, Reardon CM, McGreal GT, Hehir DJ, Kirwan WO, Brady MP. Deliberate ingestion of foreign bodies by institutionalised psychiatric hospital patients and prison inmates. *Ir J Med Sci.* 1996 Oct-Dec;165(4):294-6.

8 ^ _a b_ Grover SC, Kim YI, Kortan PP, Marcon NE. Endoscopic removal of eight gastric foreign bodies ingested sequentially in twelve days: a case of creative endoscopy. Abstract presented at *World Congress of Gastroenterology*, Montreal, Canada, September 2005.

9^ _a b_ Aoyagi, K; Maeda, K; Morita, I; Eguchi, K; Nishimura, H; Sakisaka, S (2003). "Endoscopic removal of a spoon from the stomach with a double-snare and balloon". *Gastrointestinal endoscopy* **57** (7): 990–1. doi:10.1067/mge.2003.266. PMID 12776067.

10^ Nandi, P; Ong, GB (1978). "Foreign body in the oesophagus: review of 2394 cases". *The British journal of surgery* **65** (1): 5–9. doi:10.1002/bjs.1800650103. PMID 623968.

11^ Chaikhouni, A; Kratz, JM; Crawford, FA (1985). "Foreign bodies of the esophagus". *The American surgeon* **51** (4): 173–9. PMID 3985482.

12 ^ Smith MT, Wong RK. Esophageal foreign bodies: types and techniques for removal. *Curr Treat Options Gastroenterol.* 2006 Feb;9(1):75-84.

13 ^ *a b* Seo, JK (1999). "Endoscopic management of gastrointestinal foreign bodies in children". *Indian journal of pediatrics* **66** (1 Suppl): S75–80. PMID 11132474.

14 ^ Chen, SC; Yu, SC; Yuan, RH; Chang, KJ (1997). "Endoscopic removal of a large gastric metallic watch with a polypectomy snare loop". *Endoscopy* **29** (9): S55–6. PMID 9476781.

15 ^ Neustater, B; Barkin, JS (1996). "Extraction of an esophageal food impaction with a Roth retrieval net". *Gastrointestinal endoscopy* **43** (1): 66–7. PMID 8903823.

16 ^ Yamauchi, K; Kobayashi, T; Shinomiya, T; Fujiwara, D; Ito, W; Onoda, T; Yozai, K; Ishii, T et al. (2001). "Device for the removal of button batteries". *Internal medicine (Tokyo, Japan)* **40** (1): 9–13. doi:10.2169/internalmedicine.40.9. PMID 11201377.

17 · ^ Kelly, FJ; Fussell, JC (2011 Aug). "Air pollution and airway disease.". *Clinical and experimental allergy : journal of the British Society for Allergy and Clinical Immunology* 41 (8): 1059–71. PMID 21623970.

18 ^ *a b c* Elward, Graham Douglas, Kurtis S. (2010). *Asthma*. London: Manson Pub. pp. 27–29. ISBN 978-1-84076-513-7.

19· ^ *a b* Rapini, Ronald P.; Bolognia, Jean L.; Jorizzo, Joseph L. (2007). *Dermatology: 2-Volume Set*. St. Louis: Mosby. ISBN 1-4160-2999-0.

20· ^ GINA 2011, p. 4

21· ^ O'Rourke ST (October 2007). "Antianginal actions of beta-adrenoceptor antagonists". *Am J Pharm Educ* 71 (5): 95. PMC 2064893. PMID 17998992.

22· ^ Covar, RA; Macomber, BA; Szefler, SJ (2005 Feb). "Medications as asthma trigers.". *Immunology and allergy clinics of North America* 25 (1): 169–90. PMID 15579370.

23· ^ *a b c d* Baxi SN, Phipatanakul W (April 2010). "The role of allergen exposure and avoidance in asthma". *Adolesc Med State Art Rev* 21 (1): 57–71, viii–ix. PMC 2975603. PMID 20568555.

24 ^ *a b* Maskell, Nick; Millar, Ann (2009). *Oxford desk reference.*. Oxford: Oxford University Press. p. 196. ISBN 9780199239122

25 ^ _a_ _b_ _c_ _d_ _e_ _f_ _g_ _h_ _i_ Sharma, S; Maycher, B; Eschun, G (May 2007). "Radiological imaging in pneumonia: recent innovations". *Current Opinion in Pulm*11^ Lowe, J. F.; Stevens, Alan (2000). *Pathology* (2nd ed.). St. Louis: Mosby. p. 197. ISBN 0-7234-3200-7.

26 ^ Lowe, J. F.; Stevens, Alan (2000). *Pathology* (2nd ed.). St. Louis: Mosby. p. 197. ISBN 0-7234-3200-7.

27 ^ _a_ _b_ _c_ _d_ _e_ _f_ _g_ _h_ _i_ _j_ _k_ _l_ _m_ _n_ _o_ _p_ _q_ _r_ _s_ _t_ _u_ _v_ _w_ _x_ Ruuskanen, O; Lahti, E; Jennings, LC; Murdoch, DR (2011-04-09). "Viral pneumonia". *Lancet* **377** (9773): 1264–75. doi:10.1016/S0140-6736(10)61459-6. PMID 21435708.

28 ^ _a_ _b_ Figueiredo LT (September 2009). "Viral pneumonia: epidemiological, clinical, pathophysiological and therapeutic aspects". *J Bras Pneumol* **35** (9): 899–906. doi:10.1590/S1806-37132009000900012. PMID 19820817.

29 ^ *Diffuse parenchymal lung disease : ... 47 tables* ([Online-Ausg.] ed.). Basel: Karger. 2007. p. 4. ISBN 978-3-8055-8153-0.

30 ^ _a_ _b_ Maskell, Nick; Millar, Ann (2009). *Oxford desk reference.*. Oxford: Oxford University Press. p. 196. ISBN 9780199239122.

31 ^ _a_ _b_ _c_ _d_ _e_ _f_ Murray and Nadel (2010). Chapter 37.

32^ *Clinical infectious diseases : a practical approach*. New York, NY [u.a.]: Oxford Univ. Press. 1999. p. 833. ISBN 978-0-19-508103-9.

33 ^ *Diffuse parenchymal lung disease : ... 47 tables* ([Online-Ausg.] ed.). Basel: Karger. 2007. p. 4. ISBN 978-3-8055-8153-0

34 · ^ _a_ _b_ _c_ _d_ _e_ _f_ _g_ _h_ _i_ _j_ Rajapaksa S, Starr M (May 2010). "Croup – assessment and management". *Aust Fam Physician* **39** (5): 280–2. PMID 20485713.

35 · ^ _a_ _b_ _c_ _d_ _e_ _f_ _g_ _h_ _i_ _j_ _k_ _l_ _m_ _n_ _o_ _p_ Everard ML (February 2009). "Acute bronchiolitis and croup". *Pediatr. Clin. North Am.* **56** (1): 119–33, x–xi. doi:10.1016/j.pcl.2008.10.007. PMID 19135584.

36 ^ _a_ _b_ _c_ _d_ _e_ _f_ _g_ _h_ _i_ _j_ _k_ _l_ _m_ _n_ _o_ _p_ _q_ _r_ _s_ Cherry JD (2008). "Clinical practice. Croup". *N. Engl. J. Med.* **358** (4): 384–91. doi:10.1056/NEJMcp072022. PMID 18216359.

37 ^ Papaioannou, V.; Terzi, I.; Dragoumanis, C.; Pneumatikos, I. (2009). "Negative-pressure acute tracheobronchial [[hemorrhage]] and pulmonary edema". *Journal of Anesthesia* **23** (3): 417–420. doi:10.1007/s00540-009-0757-0. Wikilink embedded in URL title (help)

38 ^ O'Leary, R.; McKinlay, J. (2011). "Neurogenic pulmonary oedema". *Continuing Education in Anaesthesia, Critical Care & Pain* **11** (3): 87–92. doi:10.1093/bjaceaccp/mkr006.

39 ^ Hampson NB, Dunford RG (1997). "Pulmonary edema of scuba divers". *Undersea Hyperb Med* **24** (1): 29–33. PMID 9068153. Retrieved 2008-09-04.

40 ^ Cochard G, Arvieux J, Lacour JM, Madouas G, Mongredien H, Arvieux CC (2005). "Pulmonary edema in scuba divers: recurrence and fatal outcome". *Undersea Hyperb Med* **32** (1): 39–44. PMID 15796313. Retrieved 2008-09-04.

41 · ^ Clark WR Jr. (1992) Smoke inhalation: diagnosis and treatment. World J Surg. 16: 24-9.

42 .^ MedlinePlus Medical Encyclopedia: Heart palpitations

43 · ^ a b c d e f g Van de Werf F, Bax J, Betriu A, *et al.* (December 2008). "Management of acute myocardial infarction in patients presenting with persistent ST-segment elevation: the Task Force on the Management of ST-Segment Elevation Acute Myocardial Infarction of the European Society of Cardiology". *Eur. Heart J.* **29** (23): 2909–45. doi:10.1093/eurheartj/ehn416. PMID 19004841.

44 ^ a b c d e Graham I, Atar D, Borch-Johnsen K, *et al.* (October 2007). "European guidelines on cardiovascular disease prevention in clinical practice: executive summary: Fourth Joint Task Force of the European Society of Cardiology and Other Societies on Cardiovascular Disease Prevention in Clinical Practice (Constituted by representatives of nine societies and by invited experts)". *Eur. Heart J.* **28** (19): 2375–414. doi:10.1093/eurheartj/ehm316. PMID 17726041..

45 · ^ Wilson PW, D'Agostino RB, Levy D, Belanger AM, Silbershatz H, Kannel WB. (1998). "Prediction of coronary heart disease using risk factor categories" (PDF). *Circulation* **97** (18): 1843–44. doi:10.1161/01.CIR.97.18.1837. PMID 9603539.

46· ^ Buse JB, Ginsberg HN, Bakris GL, *et al.* (January 2007). "Primary prevention of cardiovascular diseases in people with diabetes mellitus: a scientific statement from the American Heart Association and the American Diabetes Association". *Circulation* **115** (1): 114–26. doi:10.1161/CIRCULATIONAHA.106.179294. PMID 17192512.

47. ^ a b c Smith SC, Allen J, Blair SN, et al. (May 2006). "AHA/ACC guidelines for secondary prevention for patients with coronary and other atherosclerotic vascular disease: 2006 update endorsed by the National Heart, Lung, and Blood Institute". *J. Am. Coll. Cardiol.* **47** (10): 2130–9. doi:10.1016/j.jacc.2006.04.026. PMID 16697342.

48. ^ Mustafic, H; Jabre, P, Caussin, C, Murad, MH, Escolano, S, Tafflet, M, Périer, MC, Marijon, E, Vernerey, D, Empana, JP, Jouven, X (2012 Feb 15). "Main air pollutants and myocardial infarction: a systematic review and meta-analysis". *JAMA: the Journal of the American Medical Association* **307** (7): 713–21. doi:10.1001/jama.2012.126. PMID 22337682.

49. ^ Yusuf S, Hawken S, Ounpuu S, Bautista L, Franzosi MG, Commerford P, Lang CC, Rumboldt Z, Onen CL, Lisheng L, Tanomsup S, Wangai P Jr, Razak F, Sharma AM, Anand SS; INTERHEART Study Investigators. (2005). "Obesity and the risk of myocardial infarction in 27,000 participants from 52 countries: a case-control study". *Lancet* **366** (9497): 1640–9. doi:10.1016/S0140-6736(05)67663-5. PMID 16271645.

50. ^ Khader YS, Rice J, John L, Abueita O. (2003). "Oral contraceptives use and the risk of myocardial infarction: a meta-analysis". *Contraception* **68** (1): 11–7. doi:10.1016/S0010-7824(03)00073-8. PMID 12878281

51. ^ "malignant hypertension" at *Dorland's Medical Dictionary*

52. ^ "Hypertensive Urgencies & Emergencies - Hypertension Drug Therapy". *Systemic Hypertension*. Armenian Health Network, Health.am. 2006. Retrieved 2007-12-02. Text " Brewster LM, MD; Michael Sutters, MD " ignored (help)

53. ^ AU Corey GR; Campbell PT; Van Trigt P; Kenney RT; O'Connor CM; Sheikh KH; Kisslo JA; Wall TC (August 1993). "Etiology of large pericardial effusions". *American Journal of Medicine* **95** (2): 209–13. doi:10.1016/0002-9343(93)90262-N. PMID 8356985. More than one of |number= and |issue= specified (help)

54. ^ Campbell PT; Li JS; Wall TC; O'Connor CM; Van Trigt P; Kenney RT; Melhus O; Corey GR (April 1995). "Cytomegalovirus pericarditis: a case series and review of the literature". *American Journal of Medical Science* **309** (4): 229–34. doi:10.1097/00000441-199504000-00009. PMID 7900747. More than one of |number= and |issue= specified (help)

55. ^ Brook I. Pericarditis caused by anaerobic bacteria.Int J Antimicrob Agents 2009; 297-300.

56. ^ "Thrombus". *MedlinePlus*. U.S. National Library of Medicine.

57. ^ *a b c d e f g h i j k l m* Donnan GA, Fisher M, Macleod M, Davis SM (May 2008). "Stroke". *Lancet* **371** (9624): 1612–23. doi:10.1016/S0140-6736(08)60694-7. PMID 18468545

58. ^ *a b c d e f g h i i k* Attia J, Hatala R, Cook DJ, Wong JG (July 1999). "The rational clinical examination. Does this adult patient have acute meningitis?". *Journal of the American Medical Association* **282** (2): 175–81. doi:10.1001/jama.282.2.175. PMID 10411200.

59. · ^ *a b c d e f g* Ginsberg L (March 2004). "Difficult and recurrent meningitis". *Journal of Neurology, Neurosurgery, and Psychiatry*. 75 Suppl 1 (90001): i16–21. doi:10.1136/jnnp.2003.034272. PMC 1765649. PMID 14978146.

60. ^ *a b c d* "Gastritis". Merck. January 2007. Retrieved 2009-01-11.

61. ^ Dajani EZ, Islam K (August 2008). "Cardiovascular and gastrointestinal toxicity of selective cyclo-oxygenase-2 inhibitors in man" (PDF). *J Physiol Pharmacol*. 59 Suppl 2: 117–33. PMID 18812633.

62. ^ *a b* Siegelbaum, Jackson (2006). "Gastritis". Jackson Siegelbaum Gastroenterolgoy. Retrieved 2008-11-18.

63. ^ "Gastritis". MayoClinic. April 13, 2007. Retrieved 2008-11-18.

64. ^ Kandulski A, Selgrad M, Malfertheiner P (August 2008). "Helicobacter pylori infection: a clinical overview". *Digestive and Liver Disease* **40** (8): 619–26. doi:10.1016/j.dld.2008.02.026. PMID 18396114.

65. ^ *a b* "Alcoholic hepatitis". Mayo Clinic.

66. ^ Barosa, R.; Ramos, L. R.; Fonseca, C.; Freitas, J. (2013). "Acute hepatitis in a young woman with systemic lupus erythematosus: A diagnostic challenge". *Case Reports* **2013**: bcr2013008591. doi:10.1136/bcr-2013-008591.

67. ^ *a b* "About Wilson Disease". Wilson Disease Association.

68. ^ de Niet A, Zaaijer HL, Ten Berge I, Weegink CJ, Reesink HW, Beuers U (2012). "Chronic hepatitis E after solid organ transplantation". *Neth J Med* **70** (6): 261–266.

69. ^ Roizen MF and Oz MC, *Gut Feelings: Your Digestive System*, pp. 175–206 in Roizen and Oz (2005)

70. ^ Koppisetti, Sreedevi; Jenigiri, Bharat; Terron, M. Pilar; Tengattini, Sandra; Tamura, Hiroshi; Flores, Luis J.; Tan, Dun-Xian; Reiter, Russel J. (2008). "Reactive Oxygen Species and the Hypomotility of the Gall Bladder as Targets for the Treatment of Gallstones with Melatonin: A Review". *Digestive Diseases and Sciences* **53** (10): 2592–603. doi:10.1007/s10620-007-0195-5. PMID 18338264.

71. ^ Ortega RM, Fernández-Azuela M, Encinas-Sotillos A, Andrés P, López-Sobaler AM (1997). "Differences in diet and food habits between patients with gallstones and controls". *Journal of the American College of Nutrition* **16** (1): 88–95. PMID 9013440. Retrieved 2010-11-06.

72. ^ Misciagna, Giovanni; Leoci, Claudio; Guerra, Vito; Chiloiro, Marisa; Elba, Silvana; Petruzzi, José; Mossa, Ascanio; Noviello, Maria R. et al. (1996). "Epidemiology of cholelithiasis in southern Italy. Part II". *European Journal of Gastroenterology & Hepatology* **8**: 585–93. doi:10.1097/00042737-199606000-00017.

73. ^ Trotman, Bruce W.; Bernstein, Seldon E.; Bove, Kevin E.; Wirt, Gary D. (1980). "Studies on the Pathogenesis of Pigment Gallstones in Hemolytic Anemia". *Journal of Clinical Investigation* **65** (6): 1301–8. doi:10.1172/JCI109793. PMC 371467. PMID 7410545.

74. ^ *Endocrine and Metabolic Disorders: Cutaneous Porphyrias*, pp. 63–220 in Beers, Porter and Jones (2006)

75. ^ Thunell S (2008). "Endocrine and Metabolic Disorders: Cutaneous Porphyrias". Whitehouse Station, New Jersey: Merck Sharp & Dohme Corporation. Retrieved 2010-11-07.

76. ^ M. A. Cahan; L. Balduf, K. Colton, B. Palacioz, W. McCartney and T. M. Farrell. "Proton pump inhibitors reduce gallbladder function". *Surgical Endoscopy* **20** (9): 1364–1367. doi:10.1007/s00464-005-0247-x. PMID 16858534.

77. ^ [a][b] Reese, GE; von Roon, AC; Tekkis, PP (2009 Jan 29). "Haemorrhoids.". *Clinical evidence* **2009**. PMID 19445775.

78. ^ [a][b][c][d][e][f][g][h][i][j][k][l][m][n][o][p][q][r][s][t][u][v][w][x][y] Lorenzo-Rivero, S (August 2009). "Hemorrhoids: diagnosis and current management". *Am Surg* **75** (8): 635–42. PMID 19725283.

79 ^ a b c d e f g h i j k l m n o p q r s Kaidar-Person, O; Person, B; Wexner, SD (2007 Jan). "Hemorrhoidal disease: A comprehensive review". *Journal of the American College of Surgeons* **204** (1): 102–17. PMID 17189119.

80 ^ a b c d e f g h i j k l m n o Schubert, MC; Sridhar, S; Schade, RR; Wexner, SD (July 2009). "What every gastroenterologist needs to know about common anorectal disorders". *World J Gastroenterol* **15** (26): 3201–9. doi:10.3748/wjg.15.3201. ISSN 1007-9327. PMC 2710774. PMID 19598294.

81 ^ a b c d e f g h i j k l m n o Beck, David (2011). *The ASCRS textbook of colon and rectal surgery* (2nd ed. ed.). New York: Springer. pp. 174–177. ISBN 9781441915818.

82 ^ National Digestive Diseases Information Clearinghouse (November 2004). "Hemorrhoids". *National Institute of Diabetes and Digestive and Kidney Diseases (NIDDK), NIH*. Retrieved 18 March 2010.

83 ^ a b c d e f g h i j k l m Eckardt AJ, Baumgart DC (January 2011). "Viral gastroenteritis in adults". *Recent Patents on Anti-infective Drug Discovery* **6** (1): 54–63. PMID 21210762.

84. ^ Segal I, Walker AR (1982). "Diverticular disease in urban Africans in South Africa". *Digestion* **24** (1): 42–6. doi:10.1159/000198773. PMID 6813167.

85. ^ a b c d Szajewska, H; Dziechciarz, P (January 2010). "Gastrointestinal infections in the pediatric population.". *Current opinion in gastroenterology* **26** (1): 36–44. doi:10.1097/MOG.0b013e328333d799. PMID 19887936.

86. ^ a b Meloni, A; Locci, D, Frau, G, Masia, G, Nurchi, AM, Coppola, RC (October 2011). "Epidemiology and prevention of rotavirus infection: an underestimated issue?". *The journal of maternal-fetal & neonatal medicine : the official journal of the European Association of Perinatal Medicine, the Federation of Asia and Oceania Perinatal Societies, the International Society of Perinatal Obstetricians* **24** (Suppl 2): 48–51. doi:10.3109/14767058.2011.601920. PMID 21749188.

87. ^ a b c d e f g Webb, A; Starr, M (April 2005). "Acute gastroenteritis in children.". *Australian family physician* **34** (4): 227–31. PMID 15861741.

88. ^ Desselberger U, Huppertz HI (January 2011). "Immune responses to rotavirus infection and vaccination and associated correlates of protection". *The Journal of Infectious Diseases* **203** (2): 188–95. doi:10.1093/infdis/jiq031. PMC 3071058. PMID 21288818.

89. ^ _a b c d e f g h i j k l m n o p q r s t_ Mandell 2010, Ch. 93

90. ^ Nyachuba, DG (May 2010). "Foodborne illness: is it on the rise?". *Nutrition Reviews* **68** (5): 257–69. doi:10.1111/j.1753-4887.2010.00286.x. PMID 20500787.

91. ^ Moudgal, V; Sobel, JD (February 2012). "*Clostridium difficile* colitis: a review.". *Hospital practice (1995)* **40** (1): 139–48. doi:10.3810/hp.2012.02.954. PMID 22406889.

92. ^ _a b_ Leonard, J; Marshall, JK, Moayyedi, P (September 2007). "Systematic review of the risk of enteric infection in patients taking acid suppression.". *The American journal of gastroenterology* **102** (9): 2047–56; quiz 2057. doi:10.1111/j.1572-0241.2007.01275.x. PMID 17509031.

93. ^ _a b c d e f g h i j k l m n o p q r s t u v w x y z_ Singh, Amandeep (July 2010). "Pediatric Emergency Medicine Practice Acute Gastroenteritis — An Update". *Emergency Medicine Practice* **7** (7)

94. ^ Wangensteen OH, Bowers WF (1937). "Significance of the obstructive factor in the genesis of acute appendicitis". *Arch Surg* **34** (3): 496–526. doi:10.1001/archsurg.1937.01190090121006.

95. ^ Pieper R, Kager L, Tidefeldt U (1982). "Obstruction of appendix vermiformis causing acute appendicitis. On of the most common causes of this is an acute viral infection which causes lymphoid hyperplasia and therefore obstruction. An experimental study in the rabbit". *Acta Chir Scand* **148** (1): 63–72. PMID 7136413.

96. ^ Hollerman J. *et al.* (1988). "Acute recurrent appendicitis with appendicolith". *Am J Emerg Med* **6** (6): 614–7.

97. ^ Jones BA, Demetriades D, Segal I, Burkitt DP (1985). "The prevalence of appendiceal fecaliths in patients with and without appendicitis. A comparative study from Canada and South Africa". *Ann. Surg.* **202** (1): 80–2. doi:10.1097/00000658-198507000-00013. PMC 1250841. PMID 2990360.

98. ^ Nitecki S, Karmeli R, Sarr MG (1990). "Appendiceal calculi and fecaliths as indications for appendectomy". *Surg Gynecol Obstet* **171** (3): 185–8. PMID 2385810.

99. ^ Arnbjörnsson E (1985). "Acute appendicitis related to faecal stasis". *Ann Chir Gynaecol* **74** (2): 90–3. PMID 2992354.

100. ^ Raahave D, Christensen E, Moeller H, Kirkeby LT, Loud FB, Knudsen LL (2007). "Origin of acute appendicitis: fecal retention in colonic reservoirs: a case control study". *Surg Infect (Larchmt)* **8** (1): 55–62. doi:10.1089/sur.2005.04250. PMID 17381397.

101. ^ Burkitt DP (1971). "The aetiology of appendicitis". *Br J Surg* **58** (9): 695–9. doi:10.1002/bjs.1800580916. PMID 4937032.

102. ^ Segal I, Walker AR (1982). "Diverticular disease in urban Africans in South Africa". *Digestion* **24** (1): 42–6. doi:10.1159/000198773. PMID 6813167.

103. ^ Arnbjörnsson E (1982). "Acute appendicitis as a sign of a colorectal carcinoma". *J Surg Oncol* **20** (1): 17–20. doi:10.1002/jso.2930200105. PMID 7078180.

104. ^ Burkitt DP, Walker AR, Painter NS (1972). "Effect of dietary fibre on stools and the transit-times, and its role in the causation of disease". *Lancet* **2** (7792): 1408–12. doi:10.1016/S0140-6736(72)92974-1. PMID 4118696.

105. ^ Adamis D, Roma-Giannikou E, Karamolegou K (2000). "Fiber intake and childhood appendicitis". *Int J Food Sci Nutr* **51** (3): 153–7. doi:10.1080/09637480050029647. PMID 10945110.

106. ^ Hugh TB, Hugh TJ (2001). "Appendicectomy--becoming a rare event?". *Med. J. Aust.* **175** (1): 7–8. PMID 11476215.

107. ^ Gear JS, Brodribb AJ, Ware A, Mann JI (1981). "Fibre and bowel transit times". *Br. J. Nutr.* **45** (1): 77–82. doi:10.1079/BJN19810078. PMID 6258626.

108 Information from WIKIPEDIA

109. ^ [a] [b] Hoppe, B; Langman, CB (2003). "A United States survey on diagnosis, treatment, and outcome of primary hyperoxaluria". *Pediatric Nephrology* **18** (10): 986–91. doi:10.1007/s00467-003-1234-x. PMID 12920626

110. ^ [a] [b] National Endocrine and Metabolic Diseases Information Service (2006). "Hyperparathyroidism (NIH Publication No. 6–3425)". *Information about Endocrine and Metabolic Diseases: A-Z list of Topics and Titles*. Bethesda, Maryland: National Institute of Diabetes and Digestive and Kidney Diseases, National Institutes of Health, Public Health Service, US Department of Health and Human Services. Retrieved 2011-07-27.

111 · · ^ National Endocrine and Metabolic Diseases Information Service (2008). "Renal Tubular Acidosis (NIH Publication No. 09–4696)". *Kidney & Urologic Diseases: A-Z list of Topics and Titles*. Bethesda, Maryland: National Institute of Diabetes and Digestive and Kidney Diseases, National Institutes of Health, Public Health Service, US Department of Health and Human Services. Retrieved 2011-07-27.

112· ^ *a b c d e* Weiss, M; Liapis, H; Tomaszewski, JE; Arend, LJ (2007). "Chapter 22: Pyelonephritis and other infections, reflux nephropathy, hydronephrosis, and nephrolithiasis". In Jennette, JC; Olson, JL; Schwartz, MM et al. *Heptinstall's Pathology of the Kidney* **2** (6th ed.). Philadelphia: Lippincott Williams & Wilkins. pp. 991–1082. ISBN 978-0-7817-4750-9.

113 · · ^ *a b c d* Moe, OW (2006). "Kidney stones: pathophysiology and medical management". *The Lancet* **367** (9507): 333–44. doi:10.1016/S0140-6736(06)68071-9. PMID 16443041. .

114 ^ *a b c d e f g h* Johri, N; Cooper B, Robertson W, Choong S, Rickards D, Unwin R (2010). "An update and practical guide to renal stone management". *Nephron Clinical Practice* **116** (3): c159–71. doi:10.1159/000317196. PMID 20606476.

115· ^ Merck Sharp & Dohme Corporation (2010). "Patient Information about Crixivan for HIV (Human Immunodeficiency Virus) Infection". *Crixivan® (indinavir sulfate) Capsules*. Whitehouse Station, New Jersey: Merck Sharp & Dohme Corporation. Retrieved 2011-07-27.

116· ^ Schlossberg, D; Samuel, R (2011). "Sulfadiazine". *Antibiotic Manual: A Guide to Commonly Used Antimicrobials* (1st ed.). Shelton, Connecticut: People's Medical Publishing House. pp. 411–12. ISBN 978-1-60795-084-4.

117· ^ Carr, MC; Prien EL Jr, Babayan RK (1990). "Triamterene nephrolithiasis: renewed attention is warranted". *Journal of Urology* **144** (6): 1339–40. PMID 2231920.

118 ^ *a b c d e f g h i j k l m n o p* Nicolle LE (2008). "Uncomplicated urinary tract infection in adults including uncomplicated pyelonephritis". *Urol Clin North Am* **35** (1): 1–12, v. doi:10.1016/j.ucl.2007.09.004. PMID 18061019.

119 ^ Amdekar, S; Singh, V, Singh, DD (2011 Nov). "Probiotic therapy: immunomodulating approach toward urinary tract infection.". *Current microbiology* **63** (5): 484–90. doi:10.1007/s00284-011-0006-2. PMID 21901556.

120 ^ a b c d e f g h Lane, DR; Takhar, SS (2011 Aug). "Diagnosis and management of urinary tract infection and pyelonephritis.". *Emergency medicine clinics of North America* **29** (3): 539–52. doi:10.1016/j.emc.2011.04.001. PMID 21782073.

121 ^ a b c d e f g Dielubanza, EJ; Schaeffer, AJ (2011 Jan). "Urinary tract infections in women.". *The Medical clinics of North America* **95** (1): 27–41. doi:10.1016/j.mcna.2010.08.023. PMID 21095409.

122^ Infectious Disease, Chapter Seven, Urinary Tract Infections from *Infectious Disease Section of Microbiology and Immunology On-line*. By Charles Bryan MD. University of South Carolina. This page last changed on Wednesday, April 27, 2011

123^ a b c d e f Bhat, RG; Katy, TA, Place, FC (2011 Aug). "Pediatric urinary tract infections.". *Emergency medicine clinics of North America* **29** (3): 637–53. doi:10.1016/j.emc.2011.04.004. PMID 21782079

124 ^ a b Eves, FJ; Rivera, N (2010 Apr). "Prevention of urinary tract infections in persons with spinal cord injury in home health care.". *Home healthcare nurse* **28** (4): 230–41. doi:10.1097/NHH.0b013e3181dc1bcb. PMID 20520263.

125 ^ "Electrical Burn Injuries." Department of Surgery, Government Medical College, Miraj and General Hospital, Sangli, Maharashtra, India. 17 August 2003. Web. 29 September 2011. <http://www.medbc.com/annals/review/vol_17/num_1/text/vol17n1p9.asp>.

126 ^ a b "Etiology." Medscape Reference. n.p. n.d. Web. 29 September 2011. <http://emedicine.medscape.com/article/433682-overview#a0102>.

127 ^ a b "Electrical Burns." Burnsurgery.org. n.p. n.d. Web. 29 September 2011. <http://www.burnsurgery.org/Modules/initial_mgmt/sec_7.htm>.

128 ^ a b c d Docking, P. "Electrical Burn Injuries." Accident and emergency nursing 7.2 (1999): 70-76. Print.

129 ^ a b c d e "What is an Electrical Burn?" Electrical Safety. n.p. n.d. Web. 29 September 2011. <http://www.electricalsafety.org/what-is-an-electrical-burn/>

130 ^ Toon, Michael H ; Maybauer, Dirk M ; Arceneaux, Lisa L ; Fraser, John F ; Meyer, Walter ; Runge, Antoinette ; Maybauer, Marc O. "Children with burn injuries--assessment of trauma, neglect, violence and abuse." Journal of injury & violence research 3.2 (2011): 98-110. Print.

131. ^ <u>a b c d e f g h i j k l m n o p q r</u> Fauci, Anthony, et al. (2008). *Harrison's Principles of Internal Medicine* (17 ed.). McGraw-Hill Professional. pp. 117–121. ISBN 978-0-07-146633-2.

132. ^ Tintinalli, Judith (2004). *Emergency Medicine: A Comprehensive Study Guide, Sixth edition*. McGraw-Hill Professional. p. 1187. ISBN 0-07-138875-3.

133^ tcloonan (September 2, 2009). "Personal Protective Equipment (PPE) Use: CBRN or Non-CBRN". *A National Dialogue for the Quadrennial Homeland Security Review*. National Academy of Public Administration. Retrieved 23 June 2010.

134^ Mason, BJ.; Heyser, CJ. (Jan 2010). "The neurobiology, clinical efficacy and safety of acamprosate in the treatment of alcohol dependence". *Expert Opin Drug Saf* **9** (1): 177–88. doi:10.1517/14740330903512943. PMID 20021295.

135. ^ Mezler M.; Müller T. (2001). "Cloning and functional expression of GABA(B) receptors from Drosophila". *European Journal of Neuroscience* **13** (3): 477–486. doi:10.1046/j.1460-9568.2001.01410.x.. PMID 11168554. Unknown parameter |author 3= ignored (help)

136. ^ Dxitoyeva S.; Dimitrijevic N.; Manev H. (2001). "Gamma-aminobutyric acid B receptor 1 mediates behavior-impairing actions of alcohol in Drosophila: adult RNA interference and pharmacological evidence". *Proceedings of the National Academy of Sciences, USA* **100** (9): 5485–5490. doi:10.1073/pnas.0830111100.PMC 154371.. PMID 12692303.

137 ^ Addolorato, G.; Leggio, L.; Ferrulli, A.; Cardone, S.; Vonghia, L.; Mirijello, A.; Abenavoli, L.; D'Angelo, C. et al. (2007). "Effectiveness and safety of baclofen for maintenance of alcohol abstinence in alcohol-dependent patients with liver cirrhosis: randomised, double-blind controlled study". *Lancet* **370** (9603): 1915–1922. doi:10.1016/S0140-6736(07)61814-5.. PMID 18068515.

138 ^ Schofield, Hugh (December 6, 2008). "France abuzz over alcoholic 'cure'". BBC News. Retrieved March 2, 2013.

139 ^ Gitlow, Stuart (1 October 2006). *Substance Use Disorders: A Practical Guide* (2nd ed.). USA: Lippincott Williams and Wilkins. pp. 52 and 103–121. ISBN 978-0-7817-6998-3.

140 ^ Ogborne, AC. (June 2000). "Identifying and treating patients with alcohol-related problems". *CMAJ* **162** (12): 1705–8. PMC 1232509. PMID 10870503.

141 ^ Soyka, M.; Rösner, S. (Nov 2008). "Opioid antagonists for pharmacological treatment of alcohol dependence – a critical review". *Curr Drug Abuse Rev* **1** (3):

142. ^ "CAGE questionnaire – screen for alcohol misuse" (PDF).

143. ^ Dhalla, S.; Kopec, JA. (2007). "The CAGE questionnaire for alcohol misuse: a review of reliability and validity studies". *Clin Invest Med* **30** (1): 33–41. PMID 17716538.

144. ^ Kenneth M. Phillips (2009-12-27). "Dog Bite Statistics". Retrieved 2010-08-06.

145. ^ Chesley LC, Annitto JE, Cosgrove RA (September 1968). "The familial factor in toxemia of pregnancy". *Obstet Gynecol* **32** (3): 303–11. PMID 5742111.

146. ^ "BestBets: Risk Factors for Ectopic Pregnancy"

147. ^ Tay JI, Moore J, Walker JJ (2000). "Ectopic pregnancy". *West J Med.* **173** (2): 131–4. doi:10.1136/ewjm.173.2.131. PMC 1071024. PMID 10924442.

148. ^ a b c d Speroff L, Glass RH, Kase NG. *Clinical Gynecological Endocrinology and Infertility, 6th Ed.* Lippincott Williams & Wilkins (1999). p. 1149ff. ISBN 0-683-30379-1.

149. ^ Bukulmez O., Yarali H., Gurgan T. (1999). "Total corporal synechiae due to tuberculosis carry a very poor prognosis following hysteroscopic synechialysis". *Human Reproduction* **14** (8): 1960–1. doi:10.1093/humrep/14.8.1960. PMID 10438408.

150. ^ a b c d e f g h Wampler SM, Llanes M (September 2010). "Common scrotal and testicular problems". *Prim. Care* **37** (3): 613–26, x. doi:10.1016/j.pop.2010.04.009. PMID 20705202.

151. ^ a b Ringdahl E, Teague L (November 2006). "Testicular torsion". *Am Fam Physician* **74** (10): 1739–43. PMID 17137004.

152. ^ "Climatic Conditions and the Risk of Testicular Torsion in Adolescent Males". Jurology.com. Retrieved 2011-09-28.

153. ^ a b c d e f g h i j k l m Cardinal, R.N. & Bullmore, E.T., *The Diagnosis of Psychosis*, Cambridge University Press, 2011, ISBN 978-0-521-16484-9

154. ^ Lesser JM, Hughes S (December 2006). "Psychosis-related disturbances. Psychosis, agitation, and disinhibition in Alzheimer's disease: definitions and treatment options". *Geriatrics* **61** (12): 14–20. PMID 17184138.

155. ^ McKeith, Ian G. (February 2002). "Dementia with Lewy bodies". *British Journal of Psychiatry* **180** (2): 144–7. doi:10.1192/bjp.180.2.144. PMID 11823325.

156. ^ Wedekind S (June 2005). "[Depressive syndrome, psychoses, dementia: frequent manifestations in Parkinson disease]". *MMW Fortschr Med* (in German) **147** (22): 11. PMID 15977623.

157. ^ Lisanby, S. H.; C. Kohler, C. L. Swanson, and R. E. Gur (January 1998). "Psychosis Secondary to Brain Tumor". *Seminars in clinical neuropsychiatry* **3** (1): 12–22. PMID 10085187.

158. ^ **(Spanish)** Rodriguez Gomez, Diego; Elvira Gonzalez Vazquez and Óscar Perez Carral (August 16–31, 2005). "Psicosis aguda como inicio de esclerosis multiple / Acute psychosis as the presenting symptom of multiple sclerosis / Psicose aguda como inicio de esclerose multipla". *Revista de Neurología* **41** (4): 255–6. PMID 16075405. Retrieved 2006-09-27.

159. ^ Evans, Dwight L.; Karen I. Mason, Jane Leserman, Russell Bauer And John Petitto (2002-02-01). "Chapter 90: Neuropsychiatric Manifestations of HIV-1 Infection and AIDS". In Kenneth L Davis, Dennis Charney, Joseph T Coyle, Charles Nemeroff. *Neuropsychopharmacology: The Fifth Generation of Progress* (5th ed.). Philadelphia: Lippincott Williams & Wilkins. pp. 1281–1301. ISBN 0-7817-2837-1. Retrieved 2006-10-16.

160. ^ Tilluckdharry, C. C.; D. D. Chaddee, R. Doon, and J. Nehall (March 1996). "A case of vivax malaria presenting with psychosis". *West Indian Medical Journal* **45** (1): 39–40. PMID 8693739.

161. ^ Fallon BA, Nields JA (November 1994). "Lyme disease: a neuropsychiatric illness". *Am J Psychiatry* **151** (11): 1571–83. PMID 7943444.

162. ^ Hess A, Buchmann J, Zettl UK, *et al.* (March 1999). "Borrelia burgdorferi central nervous system infection presenting as an organic schizophrenialike disorder". *Biol. Psychiatry* **45** (6): 795. doi:10.1016/S0006-3223(98)00277-7. PMID 10188012.

163. ^ van den Bergen HA, Smith JP, van der Zwan A (October 1993). "[Lyme psychosis]". *Ned Tijdschr Geneeskd* (in Dutch; Flemish) **137** (41): 2098–100. PMID 8413733.

164. ^ Kararizou E, Mitsonis C, Dimopoulos N, Gkiatas K, Markou I, Kalfakis N (May-Jun 2006). "Psychosis or simply a new manifestation of neurosyphilis?". *J. Int. Med. Res.* **34** (3): 335–7. PMID 16866029.

165. ^ Brooke D, Jamie P, Slack R, Sulaiman M, Tyrer P (October 1987). "Neurosyphilis—a treatable psychosis". *Br J Psychiatry* **151** (4): 556. doi:10.1192/bjp.151.4.556. PMID 3447677.

166. ^ Hermle L, Becker FW, Egan PJ, Kolb G, Wesiack B, Spitzer M (1997). "[Metachromatic leukodystrophy simulating schizophrenia-like psychosis]". *Der Nervenarzt* (in German) **68** (9): 754–8. doi:10.1007/s001150050191. PMID 9411279.

167. ^ Black DN, Taber KH, Hurley RA (2003). "Metachromatic leukodystrophy: a model for the study of psychosis". *The Journal of neuropsychiatry and clinical neurosciences* **15** (3): 289–93. doi:10.1176/appi.neuropsych.15.3.289. PMID 12928504.free full text

168. ^ Kumperscak HG, Paschke E, Gradisnik P, Vidmar J, Bradac SU (2005). "Adult metachromatic leukodystrophy: disorganized schizophrenia-like symptoms and postpartum depression in 2 sisters". *Journal of psychiatry & neuroscience : JPN* **30** (1): 33–6. PMC 543838. PMID 15644995.

169. ^ Sethi NK, Robilotti E, Sadan Y (2005). "Neurological Manifestations Of Vitamin B-12 Deficiency". *The Internet Journal of Nutrition and Wellness* **2** (1).

170. ^ Masalha R, Chudakov B, Muhamad M, Rudoy I, Volkov I, Wirguin I (September 2001). "Cobalamin-responsive psychosis as the sole manifestation of vitamin B_{12} deficiency". *Isr. Med. Assoc. J.* **3** (9): 701–3. PMID 11574992.

171. ^ [a] [b] [c] [d] [e] [f] [g] [h] Herndon D (ed.). "Chapter 4: Prevention of Burn Injuries". *Total burn care* (4th ed.). Edinburgh: Saunders. p. 46. ISBN 978-1-4377-2786-9.

172. ^ [a] [b] [c] [d] [e] [f] [g] [h] [i] [j] [k] [l] [m] [n] [o] [p] [q] [r] [s] [t] [u] [v] [w] [x] [y] [z] [aa] [ab] [ac] [ad] [ae] [af] [ag] [ah] [ai] [aj] [ak] [al] [am] [an] [ao] [ap] Tintinalli, Judith E. (2010). *Emergency Medicine: A Comprehensive Study Guide (Emergency Medicine (Tintinalli))*. New York: McGraw-Hill Companies. pp. 1374–1386. ISBN 0-07-148480-9.

173. ^ [a] [b] Hardwicke, J; Hunter, T; Staruch, R; Moiemen, N (2012 May). "Chemical burns--an historical comparison and review of the literature.". *Burns : journal of the International Society for Burn Injuries* **38** (3): 383–7. PMID 22037150.

174. ^ [a] [b] [c] [d] [e] [f] [g] [h] [i] [j] [k] [l] [m] Herndon D (ed.). "Chapter 3: Epidemiological, Demographic, and Outcome Characteristics of Burn Injury". *Total burn care* (4th ed.). Edinburgh: Saunders. p. 23. ISBN 978-1-4377-2786-9

175. ^ Edlich, RF; Farinholt, HM; Winters, KL; Britt, LD; Long WB, 3rd (2005). "Modern concepts of treatment and prevention of lightning injuries.". *Journal of long-term effects of medical implants* **15** (2): 185–96. PMID 15777170.

176. ^ Prahlow, Joseph (2010). *Forensic pathology for police, death investigators, and forensic scientists*. Totowa, N.J.: Humana. p. 485. ISBN 978-1-59745-404-9.

177 ^ "Surgical Neck Fractures of the Humerus - Wheeless' Textbook of Orthopaedics". Retrieved 2007-08-16.

178 ^ "Anatomic Neck Fracture of Humerus - Wheeless' Textbook of Orthopaedics". Retrieved 2007-08-16.

179 ^ Bennett's fracture-subluxation at GPnotebook

180. ^ Hunter, Tim B; Leonard F Peltier, Pamela J Lund (May 2000). "Musculoskeletal Eponyms: Who Are Those Guys?". *RadioGraphics* **20** (3): 819–836. PMID 10835130. Retrieved 2009-10-17.

181. ^ Mellick LB, Milker L, Egsieker E (October 1999). "Childhood accidental spiral tibial (CAST) fractures". *Pediatr Emerg Care* **15** (5): 307–9. doi:10.1097/00006565-199910000-00001. PMID 10532655.

182. ^ Tim B Hunter, Leonard F Peltier, Pamela J Lund (2000). "Musculoskeletal Eponyms: Who Are Those Guys?". *RadioGraphics* **20**: 829. Retrieved 2009-11-13.

183. ^ Perry, CR; Rice S, Rao A, Burdge R. (Oct 1983). "Posterior fracture-dislocation of the distal part of the fibula. Mechanism and staging of injury". *J Bone Joint Surg Am.* **65** (8): 1149–57. PMID 6630259. Retrieved 2009-10-10.

184. ^ TheFreeDictionary > Lisfranc's fracture Citing: Mosby's Medical Dictionary, 8th edition. Copyright 2009

185 ^ Young, JW; Resnik, CS (1990 Dec). "Fracture of the Pelvis: Current Concepts of Classification". *AJR. American journal of roentgenology* **155** (6): 1169–75. PMID 2122661.

186 ^ Lee, C; Porter, K (2007 Feb). "The prehospital management of pelvic fractures.". *Emergency medicine journal : EMJ* **24** (2): 130–3. PMID 17251627.

187 ^ "Anteroposterior Compression Fracture of Pelvis (Open Book Fracture)". Elsevier: Netter's Images.

188 ^ Rothenberger, D; Velasco, R; Strate, R; Fischer, RP; Perry JF, Jr (1978 Mar). "Open pelvic fracture: a lethal injury.". *The Journal of trauma* **18** (3): 184–7. PMID 642044.

189. ^ a b Zentani A, Burslem J (December 2009). "Towards evidence based emergency medicine: best BETs from the Manchester Royal Infirmary. BET 4: use of litmus paper in chemical eye injury". *Emerg Med J* **26** (12): 887. doi:10.1136/emj.2009.086124. PMID 19934140.

190. ^ a b c d Hodge C, Lawless M (July 2008). "Ocular emergencies". *Aust Fam Physician* **37** (7): 506–9. PMID 18592066.

191. ^ Zadik Y, Sandler V, Bechor R, Salehrabi R (August 2008). "Analysis of factors related to extraction of endodontically treated teeth". *Oral Surg Oral Med Oral Pathol Oral Radiol Endod* **106** (5): e31–5. doi:10.1016/j.tripleo.2008.06.017. PMID 18718782.

192. ^ a b Hollins, Carole (2008). *Levison's Textbook for Dental Nurses*. ISBN 978-1-4051-7557-9

192. ^ a b c d Marx, John (2010). *Rosen's emergency medicine: concepts and clinical practice* (7th ed.). Philadelphia, Pennsylvania: Mosby/Elsevier. Chapter 30. ISBN 978-0-323-05472-0.

193. ^ a b Acerra JR. "Pharyngitis". *eMedicine*. Retrieved 28 April 2010.

194. ^ a b Bisno AL (January 2001). "Acute pharyngitis". *N Engl J Med* **344** (3): 205–11. doi:10.1056/NEJM200101183440308. PMID 11172144.

195. ^ "UpToDate Inc.". (registration required)

196. ^ Reynolds SC, Chow AW (2009 Sep-Oct). "Severe soft tissue infections of the head and neck: a primer for critical care physicians". *Lung* **187** (5): 271–9. doi:10.1007/s00408-009-9153-7. PMID 19653038.

197. ^ Bansal A, Miskoff J, Lis RJ (2003 Jan). "Otolaryngologic critical care". *Crit Care Clin* **19** (1): 55–72. doi:10.1016/S0749-0704(02)00062-3. PMID 12688577.

198. ^ "Mirapex product insert" (PDF). Boehringer Ingelheim. 2009. Retrieved 2010-06-30.

199. ^ "Mosby's Medical Dictionary, 8th edition". Elsevier. 2009. Retrieved 2010-06-30.

200 ^ Unless otherwise specified, reference is: Table 20-5 in Mitchell, Richard Sheppard; Kumar, Vinay; Abbas, Abul K.; Fausto, Nelson. *Robbins Basic Pathology*. Philadelphia: Saunders. ISBN 1-4160-2973-7. 8th edition.

201 ^ Sattar N, Preiss, D, Murray, HM, Welsh, P, Buckley, BM, de Craen, AJ, Seshasai, SR, McMurray, JJ, Freeman, DJ (February 2010). "Statins and risk of incident diabetes: a collaborative meta-analysis of randomised statin trials". *The Lancet* **375** (9716): 735–42. doi:10.1016/S0140-6736(09)61965-6. PMID 20167359.

202 · ^ *a b c* Table 20-7 in: Mitchell, Richard Sheppard; Kumar, Vinay; Abbas, Abul K.; Fausto, Nelson. *Robbins Basic Pathology*. Philadelphia: Saunders. ISBN 1-4160-2973-7. 8th edition.

203· ^ Thomas A Wilson, MD (2007). "Adrenal Insufficiency". *Adrenal Gland Disorders*.

204· ^ Thomas A Wilson, MD (1999). *Adrenoleukodystrophy*.

NOTES

NOTES

NOTES